SARS in China

SPONSORED BY

the Fairbank Center for East Asian Research, Harvard University,

AND BY

the Michael Crichton Fund, Harvard Medical School

SARS in China

Prelude to Pandemic?

Edited by

ARTHUR KLEINMAN

JAMES L. WATSON

STANFORD UNIVERSITY PRESS

Stanford, California 2006

Stanford University Press
Stanford, California

Library of Congress Cataloging-in-Publication Data

SARS in China : prelude to pandemic? / edited by Arthur Kleinman and James L. Watson.
p. cm.
Includes bibliographical references and index.
ISBN 0-8047-5313-X (cloth : alk. paper) —
ISBN 0-8047-5314-8 (pbk. : alk. paper)
1. SARS (Disease)—China. I. Kleinman, Arthur. II. Watson, James L.
RA644.S17S275 2005
614.5'92'00951—dc22 2005021276

Original Printing 2006
Last figure below indicates year of this printing:
15 14 13 12 11 10 09 08 07 06

Typeset at Stanford University Press in 10/15 Minion

Contents

Preface

This book is the result of a conference funded by the Fairbank Center for East Asian Research at Harvard University and held at the Kennedy School of Government in early September 2003. Funding was also provided by the Michael Crichton Fund, Department of Social Medicine, Harvard Medical School. The editors give special thanks to the director of the Fairbank Center, Wilt Idema, for his willingness to fund this project on short notice—in the immediate aftermath of the SARS crisis.

Many people helped to bring this book to publication. Muriel Bell, senior editor at Stanford University Press, attended the conference and helped us focus on the wider implications of the epidemic. Jun Jing, professor of anthropology at Tsing Hua University in Beijing, made important interventions during the conference; his ideas and suggestions enliven several of the essays in this book. Peter Benson, anthropology Ph.D. candidate at Harvard, served as our chief researcher; Wen Hao Tien, staff associate at the Fairbank Center, was flawless in her attention to detail as conference organizer. Marianne Fritz, Marilyn Goodrich, and Lynnette Simon provided vital assistance as copyeditors and project managers.

Finally, we thank our contributors for their willingness to participate in this unusual project on such short notice—less than two months in some cases. This is warp speed for academic conferences, most of which require at least a year or two of preparation and planning.

This book is transdisciplinary in a completely unselfconscious, organic sense. Contributors understood from the outset that SARS was a global crisis that defied conventional modes of analysis. The editors made an early decision *not* to round up the usual suspects for a standard academic conference. We included health-care professionals, a journalist, and a WHO representative—many of whom found themselves in the vanguard of the SARS battle. Their vivid, firsthand accounts encouraged other contributors (economists, political scientists, anthropologists) to push beyond the boundaries of their respective disciplines and write for the widest possible audience.

SARS scared the hell out of everyone associated with this project. We hope that our book will be put to practical use—in ways that we cannot anticipate—by people who find themselves in the firing line of the next global epidemic.

Cambridge, Massachusetts A.K. and J.L.W.

Contributors

ERIK ECKHOLM is a reporter for the *New York Times* and was the paper's Beijing bureau chief from 1998 to 2003.

JOAN KAUFMAN is director of the AIDS Public Policy Training Program at Harvard's Kennedy School of Government and lecturer in social medicine, Harvard Medical School. She is also senior scientist, Schneider Institute for Health Policy, Brandeis University.

ARTHUR KLEINMAN is Sidney Rabb Professor of Anthropology (Faculty of Arts and Sciences) and professor of medical anthropology and psychiatry, Harvard Medical School, Harvard University.

DOMINIC LEE is professor, Department of Psychiatry, Chinese University of Hong Kong.

SING LEE is professor, Department of Psychiatry, Chinese University of Hong Kong.

MEGAN MURRAY is assistant professor of epidemiology, Harvard School of Public Health, and an infectious disease physician at Massachusetts General Hospital, Boston.

THOMAS G. RAWSKI is professor of economics and history and University Center for International Studies Research Professor, University of Pittsburgh.

TONY SAICH is Daewoo Professor of International Affairs, Kennedy School of Government, Harvard University.

ALAN SCHNUR served as team leader, Communicable Disease Control, World Health Organization, Beijing Office.

JAMES L. WATSON is Fairbank Professor of Chinese Society and professor of Anthropology, Harvard University.

YUN KWOK WING is professor of psychiatry at the Chinese University of Hong Kong.

HONG ZHANG is assistant professor of anthropology, Colby College.

SARS in China

Introduction

SARS in Social and Historical Context

ARTHUR KLEINMAN AND JAMES L. WATSON

The SARS, or severe acute respiratory syndrome, epidemic of 2003 was one of the most dangerous health crises of our times. Although, amazingly, it lasted only a few months, the SARS epidemic rallied health specialists, journalists, and government officials on an unprecedented scale. It also raised important questions about the role of national sovereignty in an increasingly interconnected world. Other epidemics have had a more substantial impact in terms of human life. AIDS killed three million in 2003, compared to under 1,000 killed by SARS. As the essays in this book make clear, even the overall economic, political, and social impact of the SARS epidemic remains debatable.

In retrospect, SARS is probably best seen as a harbinger of future events that might be catastrophic for the global system as we know it today. Other "new" diseases, such as avian (bird) flu, threaten dire consequences—as the World Health Organization (WHO) has been quick to point out.[1] However, SARS need not be the prelude to something far worse if governments and public health agencies learn from the events of 2003. This book thus has a didactic agenda with the broadest possible policy implications: Can we avoid the Big One?

Background: Outbreak and Containment

The media coverage generated by SARS was tremendous. But we must also situate this disease in the context of popular fears, uncertainties, and social stigma, as well as within the historical framework of epidemics and infectious diseases in China, global economic and political processes, and the emergence of "new" nationalisms and competing modernities in East Asia. The various essays collected here provide a manifold perspective on SARS as a mode of "social suffering," that is, an illness experience and trauma event affecting huge numbers of people. SARS transformed, if only temporarily, the ordinary routines and rhythms of everyday life—raising the specter of massive disorder and political breakdown. The local responses evident in (among other places) Hong Kong and Beijing were as much a consequence of the global reaction to SARS as a reaction to the infection itself.[2]

The SARS epidemic emerged in social conditions already undergoing rapid change and in a political environment rife with uncertainty. The entire regional economy of East Asia was slowly recovering from the collapse of 1997; the public panic generated by SARS further undermined local economies. The skittishness was palpable: months after the epidemic had "ended," a single case in Singapore (a medical technician who contracted SARS in the course of his lab work) sent financial markets in East Asia plummeting.[3] In the years immediately preceding the outbreak, China's urban centers were inundated with migrants from the countryside who were far too numerous for effective biopolitical control of the kind imposed during the Maoist era.[4] Furthermore, the growing specter of a potential HIV/AIDS crisis in China conditioned public responses to SARS.[5]

Over the past two decades, the global HIV/AIDS epidemic has encouraged public health authorities to become increasingly interested in the private lives and behaviors of patients. The intimacies of biosocial knowledge thus provided a unique idiom through which illness experiences could be publicized, but also produced powerful forms of social stigma—based on perceived notions of moral or social deviance. The monitoring process often compounded the suffering of disease victims and undermined effective treatment. In short, the targets of biomedical scrutiny had every incentive to avoid health officials.

SARS, too, prompted an urgent "desire to know." Only in this case, health-care professionals themselves bore much of the social stigma associated with SARS, and the taint of the disease affected their families and friends in an ever-widening circle of suspicion (see chapters 7 and 9). The HIV/AIDS struggles demonstrate the urgent need for integration and communication across various fields of medicine, as well as heightened sensitivities to the human dimensions of illness, suffering, and healing.[6]

These issues reemerged during the SARS epidemic and are addressed, in one way or another, in the chapters that follow. The most obvious parallel between SARS and the handling of previous global epidemics is the way in which social experiences were shaped by rational bureaucratic language, biomedical knowledge, and political ideologies.[7] In many respects, China's handling of SARS reflected "archaic" modes of governance: mass mobilization, authoritarian control from the center, and the uncompromising use of military and police power (see chapter 3). In April 2003, no one was certain where SARS would lead: Would it become a worldwide disaster with high lethality on the order of the 1918 influenza pandemic? In China, this would have meant widespread death, economic paralysis, and political chaos—conditions that recall historical episodes of dynastic collapse and succession to new regimes.

The public health infrastructure was in fact overwhelmed, according to James Maguire, the leader of a CDC team that traveled in China monitoring the progress of the disease. Chinese officials and international experts were visibly shaken by the crisis and worried that the final outcome might ultimately be disastrous. Detainees in Beijing hospitals were escaping, because rates of transmission were higher in clinical contexts than on the streets. The escapes ended abruptly when security forces were stationed in and around hospitals.[8]

Much of this was rightly blamed on the Chinese government, which at the early stages of the epidemic withheld information, controlled the media, and discouraged international access to SARS victims. China's central leadership, headed by the recently installed President and General Secretary Hu Jintao and Premier Wen Jiabao, fired two key figures, the minister of health and the mayor of Beijing, who immediately became scapegoats for government blunders. Then, in what can only be described as an amazing reversal, after implementing draconian techniques that could never be deployed in democratic societies, China emerged as a paragon of public health responsibility.[9] "The international loss of face and China's dramatic policy reversal after April 20, 2003, set in motion the actions that brought SARS under control," Joan Kaufman writes in chapter 3.

> What happened next is a global lesson in how political will and national mobilization are required for tackling serious threats to public health, and provides important lessons for China's long overdue response to its growing epidemics of AIDS, tuberculosis, and hepatitis. China's extensive health infrastructure, albeit weakened by years of underinvestment, rose to the occasion once China's national leadership provided the mandate for action. Few countries in the world have China's capacity for national mobilization, which extends to the remotest corners of this large and increasingly independent nation.

An important turning point was the May 1, 2003, national holiday weekend. The Chinese government cancelled the holiday—under any other circumstances an almost unimaginable political action—to prevent interregional travel. Any school or hospital that had at least one confirmed case of SARS was quarantined. A 1,000-bed quarantine facility was constructed in Beijing; work continued twenty-four hours a day, and the project was completed in less than a week. Other hospitals were converted to handle infectious disease patients. James Maguire, chief of parasitic diseases at the Centers for Disease Control (CDC), reports that 5,327 cases of SARS were treated in China, with at least 349 known deaths.[10]

Based on observations at Beijing hospitals in May, Maguire reports that the success of infection control was due in large part to the dedication and determination of nurses and doctors who worked under life-threatening circumstances. Medical and public health students, out of school because of the holiday, were stationed in the wards to monitor the micro-procedures of hygiene and treatment, thus ensuring that health-care workers did not transmit infection across patients or among themselves.[11]

By the end of May, the spread of SARS had been effectively controlled. Confirmed cases were accounted for and quarantined in hospitals. The epidemic had peaked and quickly waned. Chinese-style intervention was extolled as a means of controlling future epidemics.

Many observers hope that the SARS experience will produce a more transparent handling of China's growing AIDS problem. This does not seem to be happening, however. Meanwhile, the winter 2004 avian flu outbreaks were subject to government cover-ups, followed by delayed control measures. China, Vietnam, and Thailand were all slow in responding to avian flu,[12] which leads one to speculate that there are larger political forces at work. When a nation's health sector threatens economic interests, government authorities are reluctant to commit themselves to costly control programs. In such cases, international pressure and WHO intervention may be the only solution.

SARS in the United States

"If the SARS outbreak has taught us anything," said Ilona S. Kickbusch of the Yale School of Public Health, "it is how interconnected the world is. . . . This isn't just an issue for developing countries. . . . When the SARS outbreak spread to Canada we saw just how close to home it really was."[13] In March 2003, with cases already being identified in Canada, the attention of U.S. health and immigration authorities shifted dramatically. The passive observation of an overseas crisis was transformed into an urgent priority almost overnight. One example highlights the magnitude and unpredictability of the threat: A student at the University of Connecticut came down with a fever after flying home from Germany. One of his fellow passengers had been a doctor who had worked recently in Singapore hospitals. The student went to classes. Public health officials identified everyone in those classes and people who had come into contact with the individual. The student tested negative.[14]

Popular fears in the United States, even in the absence of large numbers of actual cases,[15] were in part caused by the general medical and epidemiological uncertainty about SARS. Experts had some idea of the potential magnitude of the threat, but this information was itself dangerous, potentially redoubling and intensifying popular fears. In April, Megan Murray of the Harvard School of Public Health (the author of chapter 1) concluded that the disease is more contagious than smallpox—with each case having the potential of infecting five other people. In a population of one million, about 900,000 could contract the illness. And with a 4 percent mortality rate, approximately 36,000 people could die. Murray concludes, "If these data were even close to correct, we could have a very serious global pandemic of SARS."[16]

During this period, popular fears also fixated on the possibility of bioterrorism and contamination of the American food supply. "The greatest fear," a *New York Times* article mused, "is that the next plague will be the equivalent of the meteorological perfect storm, possibly from an untreatable respiratory infection that spreads rapidly."[17] The specter of worldwide catastrophe, fed no doubt by Hollywood films and popular thrillers, helps frame current perceptions of future epidemics—views that build on incomplete knowledge of disease transmission.

It is not surprising that stringent precautions were quickly established to identify and manage potential SARS cases in the United States. In April 2003, for example, Harvard University placed a moratorium on university-sponsored or university-related travel to China, Hong Kong, Singapore, Taiwan, Vietnam, and Toronto, Canada, saying: "University funds will not be used to support trips . . . nor will the University facilitate or otherwise endorse travel to these areas until further notice."[18] The ban was lifted for Canada in May, but destinations in Asia remained on the list through the summer of 2003. Students who defied this warning faced a ten-day suspension upon their return. Harvard's policy reflected the general positions taken by other American institutions, including business corporations, nonprofit organizations, and government agencies. SARS loomed large in the American imagination during the winter of 2002 and spring of 2003.

The History of Epidemics and Infectious Disease in China

Until the early twentieth century, there was no clear separation between curative and preventative medicine in China.[19] There was, however, what might be called a "high-order medical system," as opposed to the various popular medical practices. The former was embedded in the Confucian tradition and supported by imperial patronage. All Chinese medical systems were oriented toward personal and family problems resulting from individual cases of illness. Epidemics were beyond the scope of conventional knowledge. Nor did healing traditions foster a means for the delivery of medical care during famines or floods.[20]

The first public vaccinations against communicable diseases in the Chinese-speaking world were carried out by the British colonial authorities in Hong Kong during the late nineteenth century.[21] Plague was common in Hong Kong between 1894 and 1924, taking a considerable toll. From May to September 1894, plague reached epidemic proportions there, killing at least 2,550 persons. Many of the sufferers were transported to Canton (Guangzhou) for treatment. Those affected were frequently abandoned, and the bodies of the dead were dumped. An official report states that the most difficult aspect of controlling the epidemic was the resistance of families to the removal of sufferers to hospitals under colonial management.[22] There was international frustration that the Chadwick report of 1883, which detailed hygienic conditions along the southern Chinese coast and the potential for an outbreak of infectious diseases, had not been taken seriously. If it had, many insisted, the epidemic would not have started.[23] At the same time, it is clear that Western medicine was no more effective than traditional Chinese medicine in treating infectious diseases.[24]

In 1931, the European Conference on Rural Hygiene, organized by the League of Nations, called the first international meeting on rural health care. The conference recommended that first priority be given to the control of infectious diseases within the broader agenda of modernizing health care in China and providing equal services for all.[25] Efficient public health interventions were based on an indigenous system of collective responsibility called *bao jia* (literally "protect families") that facilitated record keeping and household registration. This *bao jia* system allowed local police to identify everyone in the community, thereby facilitating not only vaccination but speedy burial of cholera victims. In some cities, streets were widened, pigs were banned in urban districts, and residents were flogged for leaving garbage in front of their houses.[26]

During the mid twentieth century, the newly established Chinese communist state attempted to combat infectious disease on a massive scale. "Prevention first" was the official slogan that guided national public health policy.[27] In 1949 (the year the Communist Party took power), a Central Plague Prevention Committee organized medical teams to combat epidemics throughout the country. The state sponsored vaccination projects, aimed mainly at eradicating smallpox and plague, as well as cholera, diphtheria, and typhoid.[28] "No other country in the world has so successfully controlled venereal diseases," writes one observer.[29]

Smallpox, which had been rampant a decade before, had been eradicated by the mid 1950s. The last outbreak was reported in March 1960 in Yunnan province.[30] William Foege's essay on "Surveillance and Antiepidemic Work," is one of the best descriptions of the operation of the rural health stations established in the 1950s.[31] He notes that the success of China's anti-epidemic programs was due to the preexisting medical system, which, "unlike that of most countries, provides a mechanism for vaccinating every person."[32] Furthermore, despite the seeming uniformity of policy at the national level, procedures and practices differed markedly at the local level.[33]

Infectious diseases remained a problem in rural areas, even as national rates were plummeting. During the Great Leap Forward (1958–60), the Ministry of Health blamed the continuing problem of infectious diseases on the "increased susceptibility of sections of the [rural] population." The staggering problems of famine and economic collapse in the countryside were only mentioned in passing.[34] Vast amounts of money were spent on pest extermination campaigns during this period, while funds for the control of communicable diseases declined.[35] Not surprisingly, serious health crises occurred and party officials found scapegoats to take the blame.[36] This was precisely what also happened during the SARS epidemic half a century later.

The Chinese government consolidated its authority during the late 1950s, partly through a series of patriotic health campaigns aimed at rectifying glaring deficiencies. On 12 January 1956, the *People's Daily* announced a nationwide campaign to eradicate the "four menaces": mosquitoes, flies, rats, and sparrows.[37] Although this movement was short-lived, in Heilongjiang that year, 200,000 youths were organized to catch pests. A year later, the minister of health at the time, Li Dequan, admitted that preventing epidemics "cannot be accomplished within a short time." Furthermore, he noted, "occasional ineffectual Patriotic Health Movements" did not help solve long-term problems.[38]

A classic example of mass mobilization focused on a disease was the 1958 campaign against venereal disease in Jiangxi province. Every social and political organization in the province was mobilized to eradicate the targeted diseases; health education was promoted via pamphlets, lectures, posters, plays, radio broadcasts, newspaper articles, and small-group discussions.[39] The campaign built on techniques used in China during in the 1930s, as well as on government programs to eliminate hookworm in the United States.[40]

Mass mobilizations of this nature had a number of political effects. First, they extended and legitimated the party's control in the Chinese countryside.[41] Second, they reinforced the authority of elite (primarily urban) medical experts and doctors.[42] The gaps between these urban-based medical elites and the less prestigious, underfunded rural health operatives were glaringly evident during the SARS epidemic.

The case of the 1942 cholera epidemic in Yunnan province, which killed nearly 200 people, provides an interesting historical parallel to the 2002–2003 SARS crisis. The public was "deeply disturbed by the epidemic and expended a tremendous amount of energy in measures to fight it." Local hospitals and schools took preventative measures and provided treatment at little or no cost; posters were plastered throughout the district describing modes of contagion. But Western medicine was not used to combat the disease.[43]

Hsu discovered that Western medical knowledge and practices did not conform to local cultural rationalities and healing methods. Hsu's rich ethnographic account points to a number of factors that are overlooked in most assessments of Chinese epidemics. First, patients reported that cholera vaccinations were painful, a view that did not encourage others to follow.[44] Second, during the Yunnan epidemic, police began monitoring streets and ensured that inhabitants kept public spaces clean.[45] This may have created tensions within the community, singling out certain districts or families as unsanitary and hence prone to contagion. Perceptions of social stigma developed very quickly in the wake of the epidemic and worked against containment. Hsu notes that "nurses even went out into the streets urging people to adopt certain preventative and curative measures; yet they found few people willing to follow these measures."[46] The force of stigma was reflected in the ritual life of the community. Early in the epidemic, elaborate funerals were organized by the families of those who died of cholera. Soon, however, funeral processions were reduced in size and ostentation to avoid public scrutiny—thus reinforcing the stigma associated with disease.[47]

Hsu argues that, in the local context, illness becomes a sign of moral contamination, just as moral behavior indexes one's potential danger as a spreader of disease.[48] Joseph Bosco's work on local efforts to control SARS in Hong Kong parallels some of Hsu's conclusions, even though the two epidemics were separated by six decades.[49]

Yuqun Liao has proposed the notion of "local disease" to describe conditions that arise within specific cultural or linguistic domains, making them difficult for foreigners to understand.[50] A local disease, as defined by Liao, blurs the division between physical illness and social imbalance, calling attention to the dialectical relations between society and cosmology. This suggests that cultural factors are crucial for understanding how epidemics are perceived. Local reactions to SARS, as outlined in chapters 7 and 9, reaffirm the value of this approach.

The Organization of the Book

Megan Murray, an epidemiologist at the Harvard School of Public Health, sets out the epidemiological parameters of the SARS epidemic in chapter 1. She places the Chinese case in global perspective and outlines the uncertainties regarding its causes. Murray's work is critical for understanding the terrifying potential of SARS. In chapter 2, Alan

Schnur, who was the leader of a WHO team in Beijing that monitored and advised the Chinese government during the epidemic, gives us an insider's perspective on the events of 2003. Schnur describes the role that WHO experts played on the ground and recounts their experiences of working with China's Ministry of Health and the political leadership. The WHO became a major player during the epidemic, thus reaffirming the organization's global role and setting the stage for future interventions.

Joan Kaufman views the SARS epidemic within the broader context of the Chinese health-care system in chapter 3. She identifies the unique features of that system and shows how the Chinese government made the transition from global pariah early in the outbreak to international hero at its terminus. Kaufman argues that rural health care in China has been systematically dismantled over the past two decades and that the current focus on fee-based financing for curative care has weakened the response to infectious disease. She provides an in-depth case study of how the SARS mobilization worked in one poor rural county. As local officials came to sense their careers hanging in the balance, economic and political resources were allocated to control SARS. The handling of the epidemic was thus rooted in control measures that underplayed individual civil liberties to serve the needs of public safety. If this program succeeded, it also exposed the deterioration of rural public health care.

The next section of the book deals with the political and economic consequences of the epidemic. Tony Saich, a close observer of Chinese politics, describes the complex and multifaceted response to SARS. Saich treats the health emergency as a window on China's new, often problematic status in the international community. Writing as a political scientist, his focus is on the higher ranks of the Chinese Communist party. Thomas Rawski, who has devoted his career to understanding the Chinese economy, cautions against overemphasizing the economic effects of SARS. He also questions the accuracy of Chinese government statistics that depict an economy experiencing steady, unparalleled growth. SARS was potentially a major threat, but the epidemic was controlled quickly enough, according to Rawski, to minimize what could have been much greater economic damage. Erik Eckholm served as *New York Times* bureau chief in Beijing during the SARS crisis, and, as such, he was in a unique position to observe the actions of Chinese government officials. In chapter 6, he describes the often-surreal events as they unfolded.

The chapters that follow examine the social and ethical effects of SARS. Dominic Lee and Yung Kwok Wing discuss the psychological impact of SARS by recounting their personal experiences as physicians in a Hong Kong clinic at the height of the epidemic. Their testimony, reproduced in chapter 7, conveys the bone-chilling terror experienced by those in the front lines of treatment. Hong Zhang surfed the Internet and spoke with her friends in China to collect examples of the gallows humor that surfaced during the SARS outbreak. Her account in chapter 8 reveals a feature of the 2003 crisis that escaped international attention but would be familiar to anyone who has lived in countries controlled by socialist regimes.

The book concludes with two essays that set the SARS epidemic in comparative, cross-cultural perspective. Arthur Kleinman and Sing Lee explore the psychological and cultural dimensions of SARS in chapter 9. They focus on the social stigma that rapidly conditioned public and personal responses to the crisis. Their analysis may help mitigate the trauma experienced by people who fall victim to future epidemics—thereby encouraging voluntary compliance with quarantine measures. James L. Watson's essay focuses on the long-term consequences of the SARS crisis and what it portends for the future of international travel and personal mobility. Watson, an anthropologist who studies local responses to globalization in Hong Kong and China, argues in chapter 10 that SARS was a warning—a wakeup call that demonstrates the inherent fragility of the global system.

Where Do We Go from Here?

Seen in the context of avian flu and the major outbreaks of flu in the twentieth century—most of which appear to have originated in south China—the SARS crisis suggests that a new approach to understanding human epidemics must be found. Virologists need to work in teams consisting of ecologists, biologists, soil scientists, economists, political scientists, demographers, epidemiologists, anthropologists, and ethicists. This is the only way we can hope to understand the intersection of ecological, social, and biological processes that underlie emergent infectious diseases. At issue here are the migration of waterfowl, the intensive cultivation of ducks, chickens, and pigs in settings of dense human habitation, trade in and sale of wild animals, the migration of workers, and the complexities of local cultural practices. The isolationist (and elitist) conventions of traditional academic disciplines make it difficult for younger scholars to engage in this type of team research. This is not a matter of funding alone. The real problem lies in reward and promotion structures that are increasingly obsolete in the twenty-first-century world. If this book accomplishes anything, we hope that our collective efforts will help promote the cause of teamwork and transdisciplinary research.

At this writing (winter 2005), avian flu has killed 46 people in Vietnam, Cambodia, and Thailand. Scientists all over the world are working—flat out—to find a vaccine for this emergent threat.[51] We can only hope that this book will be the record of an isolated biosocial event, a historical curiosity that will not be repeated in the twenty-first century.

PART I

The Epidemiological and Public Health Background

CHAPTER ONE

The Epidemiology of SARS

MEGAN MURRAY

In mid November 2002, a middle-aged businessman from Foshan, China, was hospitalized for an atypical pneumonia. He eventually recovered from his illness, although not before infecting four of his health-care attendants. Later, this patient would be recognized as the first detected case of SARS in the world.

Little concrete information about the spread of the disease emerged from China over the next few months, but in mid February, the World Health Organization was notified of an outbreak of a respiratory illness involving 305 cases and causing 5 deaths in Guangdong province. Even at the time of this report, it was clear that many of the cases had occurred among the health-care workers who had cared for infected patients. What was not apparent until much later was that food handlers working in Guangdong's busy markets were also heavily represented among those who became ill with the mysterious illness.

This was not the first time a new respiratory infection had emerged from southern China. In 1957, a new strain of influenza appeared in Hunan, China, which spread throughout the world and led to the Asian flu pandemic of that year. That strain persisted until 1968, when it was supplanted by yet another influenza strain that emerged from southern China and rapidly moved to Hong Kong before disseminating around the globe. Since then, several new variants of flu have arisen from the same region, most recently, an avian strain of influenza A that emerged in 1997, killing large numbers of poultry before it spread to humans, and that resulted in at least six deaths among the eighteen cases reported. Despite fears that this highly virulent avian strain might lead to a worldwide pandemic, there was fortunately no person-to-person spread of this virus. All of those who became ill had some connection with the live chicken markets in Hong Kong, and no further human cases were reported after influenza was brought under control in its avian host through mass slaughter of poultry.

With the last three influenza pandemics all originating in southern China, many researchers have wondered why this area has been the breeding-ground from which these new virus strains have emerged. Influenza A is widespread in nature and can be found in a range of animal hosts, including birds and pigs. Most influenza researchers believe that avian strains of influenza A acquire mutations that enable them to cross the species barrier and go on to infect humans and then spread among them. Although these mutations are rare events, southern China is home to an enormous poultry industry; the sheer numbers of birds on these farms means that there is ample opportunity for the population of viruses to grow and for one of these multitudinous virus strains to undergo a rare mutation.

Given this history, the Chinese authorities immediately suspected that a new influenza strain was the most likely culprit responsible for the mysterious respiratory infection spreading in Guangdong. However, tests for influenza quickly came back negative. Given recent events in other parts of the world, the Chinese also sought and ruled out suspected agents of bio-terrorism such as anthrax and plague, organisms that can cause respiratory symptoms. To complicate matters further, several different common and not so common respiratory pathogens were found in the respiratory secretions of at least some of the infected;

these organisms included human meta-pneumovirus and chlamydia, a relatively common cause of atypical pneumonia among young people worldwide.

All of this remained a fairly local problem until February 21, 2003, the day on which a 65-year-old physician from Guangdong checked into a room on the ninth floor of the Metropole Hotel in Hong Kong, already symptomatic with the infection for which he had been treating people back at home. Although the doctor had little contact with others in the hotel, twelve guests staying on the same floor were eventually diagnosed with SARS. Among them were a Chinese businessman who traveled on to Hanoi to become the index case of the outbreak there, a Singaporean woman who was hospitalized soon after her return to her native city, an elderly woman from Toronto who went home to expose her large family in Canada, and a group of others who were admitted to Hong Kong hospitals, where they spread the disease to many of the hospital staff to whom they were exposed. Another one of these cases was a young man who was treated for a week in a Hong Kong hospital with a jet nebulizer that aerosolized his respiratory secretions, thus disseminating the virus throughout the hospital environment.

Although it was not clear how these people became infected at the Metropole Hotel when they had no direct contact with the doctor, it was clear that this cosmopolitan setting had provided the opportunity for the virus to infect travelers who would go on to spread the disease throughout the world. Through this seeding, subsequent local epidemics occurred in Hanoi, Singapore, Toronto, and Hong Kong with transmission to hospital staff and patients a major route of subsequent spread. The Singaporean woman was ultimately linked to over 100 cases of SARS in Singapore and the elderly resident of Toronto initiated the Scarborough Grace Hospital cluster that involved 132 people and caused 12 deaths.

By mid March, SARS had spread to seven countries, and by late

March, 1,320 cases and 50 deaths had been reported. On March 30, 2003, Hong Kong officials announced that a large cluster of cases had occurred almost simultaneously in a huge housing complex known as the Amoy Gardens. Up to this point, transmission appeared to have occurred principally through the respiratory route, but the Amoy Gardens outbreak now raised the possibility that environmental transmission might also play a key role. An investigation conducted by the Hong Kong authorities identified a faulty sewage system as the probable means of spread of the virus in the building complex. The initial case was identified as a man being treated for kidney disease at a large Hong Kong hospital, who had developed symptoms of SARS while he was visiting his brother at the apartment complex. As reported by the WHO, subsequent rapid spread to 321 other residents is thought to have involved "defective U-traps [or P traps] in bathrooms, an amplifying effect of bathroom exhaust fans, a cracked sewer vent pipe serving Block E, and an aerodynamic effect in a lightwell to which bathroom windows opened" (www.who.int/csr/don/2003_04_18/en/ [accessed 23 March 2005]).

Over the next few months, newspapers throughout the world were filled with daily reports on the spread of SARS; some of the news was good, but much of it was bad. By late April, SARS had been successfully contained in Vietnam and was beginning to taper off in Singapore, Hong Kong, and Toronto. In the meantime, however, the epidemic had taken off in Taiwan after the diagnosis was initially missed in a patient who subsequently visited multiple clinics and hospitals, spreading infection widely. The stringent control measures taken by various countries throughout Asia have been well described in the media—these included the closing of schools, widespread screening for fever in airports and at other checkpoints for travelers, the strict isolation of infected cases and the quarantining of those exposed to known cases. Since the implementation of these control measures coincided with the decline in cases, most public health authorities have concluded that these interventions had a major impact on controlling the disease and eventually led to its elimination. By the end of the epidemic, more than 8,000 cases had been reported, and there had been 916 deaths.

Although the end of the epidemic brought an enormous sense of relief to the many people whose lives had been impacted by it, investigators who were trying to understand its origin and develop future safeguards against SARS had little respite. For epidemiologists who study the patterns of disease spread in communities, the occurrence of a new infectious disease raises a number of preeminent questions for the epidemiologist, many of which have still not been adequately answered:

Where did it come from?
By what routes does it spread?
How transmissible is it?
What needs to be done to contain it?
How virulent is it?
Will it return?

Where Did SARS Come From?

In order to determine where SARS came from, it would first be necessary to identify the infectious agent. Despite the initial misidentification of the organism as chlamydia, this was accomplished amazingly quickly; by the third week in March, several different research groups in various countries had identified a novel coronavirus from the secretions of SARS patients, which was named SARS-CoV.[1,2] The coronaviruses are a diverse group of RNA viruses that cause respiratory and gastrointestinal diseases in humans and other animals. The prefix "corona" refers to the crownlike appearance produced by projections from the surface of the virions when viewed through an electron microscope. These projections represent "spike" or "S" proteins, which bind to the host cellular receptors allowing the viruses to enter host cells. There are three distinct groups of coronaviruses; groups 1 and 2 contain mammalian viruses, whereas group 3 consists only of avian pathogens. Specific coronaviruses usually have a narrow host range, meaning that each type of virus only infects its natural host or closely related species and is not transmissible across the species barrier. Animal coronaviruses can cause serious illness, and some coronaviruses, such as infectious bronchitis virus (IBV) of chickens, have had a major economic impact on the poultry industry. By contrast, until SARS emerged, human coronaviruses were responsible for about 30 percent of colds but had never previously been associated with severe respiratory disease or death.

Soon after the organism had been identified, complete genome sequences were published and compared to genomic data from other known coronaviruses.[3,4] SARS was not found to be closely related to any of these viruses and, indeed, was so dissimilar to previously described viruses that it could not be placed in any one of the three groups of coronaviruses. This finding led to headlines such as this one:

> Is SARS from Mars? UK scientists say maybe. Could SARS have come from Mars? Or elsewhere in the vast reaches of outer space? Unlikely, say earthbound microbiologists. But some scientists from the United Kingdom aren't so sure.

The UK scientists referred to were a group that included professors from the Cardiff Center for Astrobiology and the Department of Molecular Biology and Biotechnology at Sheffield University, who wrote a letter to the highly respected medical journal the *Lancet* saying that "the virus is unexpectedly novel and appeared without warning in mainland China. A small amount of the culprit virus introduced into the stratosphere could make a first tentative fallout east of the great mountain range of the Himalayas, where the stratosphere is thinnest . . . the subsequent course of its global progress will depend on stratospheric transport and mixing, leading to a fall out continuing seasonally over a few years."[5]

Nonetheless, when earthbound scientists looked for the newly described coronavirus in the marketplaces of Guangdong, they found a very closely related virus in masked palm civets and raccoon dogs in a live animal market. Although this does not provide direct evidence that these animals were the source of SARS—they may in fact have been infected by humans rather than vice versa—it does suggest that the species barrier had been breached, a finding supported by the ease with which SARS-CoV infected a range of cell lines from different species in vitro.

While this species-hopping may be unusual behavior for a coronavirus, it is certainly not an uncommon event for other pathogens. Several months after the advent of SARS, a small outbreak of monkeypox among humans was reported in the United States, and the cases were traced to a shipment of Gambian giant rats imported from Ghana and sold as pets.[6] Monkeypox is a viral infection very similar to smallpox, although causing a less virulent illness. Most of the cases in the United States were thought to have spread directly from animals to humans, although some human-to-human transmission is known to occur, and it could not be ruled out in cases in which multiple household members became infected. What makes SARS different from monkeypox and the host of other diseases that cross from animals to humans is that, unlike these zoonoses, SARS was readily transmitted from person to person after the initial introduction from another species. Although monkeypox may occasionally be transmitted from person to person, it is relatively inefficient at this type of spread and the transmission chain soon dies out.

By What Routes Does SARS Spread?

Clearly, SARS spread rapidly from person to person, particularly among close contacts and health-care workers who cared for SARS patients. It is also clear that the predominant mode of transmission was through respiratory secretions, as with most respiratory infections. Most infectious disease epidemiologists recognize two distinct patterns of respiratory transmission: that due to the aerosolization of small infectious particles that then remain suspended in air, ready to be inhaled into the lungs of those re-breathing that air; and that due to larger respiratory droplets that are projected short distances through sneezes or coughs or via the intermediary of hands. Organisms that can be aerosolized pose a greater threat in terms of transmission capacity, since simple barrier measures that prevent exposure to respiratory droplets will not protect one from inhaling contaminated air. The little evidence available to date suggests that SARS may be spread predominantly through large respiratory droplets and is thus only spread over short distances. These data come from hospital studies that sought to determine risk factors for infection among health-care workers exposed to SARS patients. In these small surveys, the wearing of protective masks and the practice of contact precautions was associated with a decrease in risk for infection, leading to the inference that transmission must occur through close contact.[7,8]

The Amoy Garden experience made it clear that respiratory transmission is not the sole route by which SARS spreads. SARS-CoV has been detected in stool and urine. Fecal shedding has been shown to last, on average, for several weeks. However, it is unclear how much, if any, transmission occurs directly through the fecal-oral or fecal-respiratory route. Nonetheless, should long-term fecal shedding occur in some infected people, this may provide a means by which SARS could be reintroduced into circulation in human communities after having apparently been eliminated.

Other routes of transmission that have been suggested include animals that have been infected by humans but then go on to infect other humans through contaminated fecal droppings. One researcher hypothesized that rats dwelling on the rooftops of the crowded Amoy Garden complex could have been the vector by which the virus spread in that environment,[9] but there has been no subsequent proof that animals have acted as vectors in the spread of the disease. If animals such as rats were infected by humans, they could serve as a reservoir in which the virus could remain undetected for a prolonged period but through which the disease might reemerge.

Another potential route by which SARS might return is through research laboratory accidents that lead to the infection of lab workers. Two such episodes have already occurred. The first involved a researcher in a Singapore virology laboratory in September 2003; the second occurred in a laboratory worker at a Taiwan military hospital in December 2003. Investigations of these laboratory-acquired cases showed that inadequate safety standards were employed in both cases and have led to a call for more rigorous monitoring of safety procedures in the many laboratories throughout the world where SARS-CoV is kept.

How Transmissible Is SARS?

Early predictions about the course of the SARS epidemic were based on limited data on the relative infectiousness of the virus compared to other known viral and bacterial pathogens. As the epidemic progressed, it became clear that SARS was less transmissible than other epidemic viral pathogens such as measles or influenza, which spread more rapidly and produce more secondary cases for each infectious person. Infectious disease epidemiologists use a measure known as the basic reproductive number, or R_0, to quantify the transmissibility of an infectious agent. R_0 is defined as the expected number of secondary infectious cases generated by an average infectious case in a population in which everyone is susceptible. This quantity determines the potential for an infectious agent to start an outbreak, the extent of transmission in the absence of control measures, and the ability of control measures to reduce spread. R_0 is the product of the average number of contacts of an infectious individual over time, the likelihood of transmission given a contact between an infectious case and a susceptible person and the mean duration of infectiousness. Although it is a highly simplified summary of a pathogen's epidemic potential, R_0 can be used to predict the outcome of an introduction of infection into a population. If $R_0 > 1$, the number of people infected will grow and an epidemic will take place. If $R_0 < 1$, we expect the disease to die out.

One way to estimate the number of people infected by a single infectious case is simply to count the number of secondary cases known to be infected by each "index" case. Data collected during the early weeks of the epidemic in Singapore suggested that the number of secondary cases per index case was relatively high during the first week of the outbreak but later fell to close to one, possibly after the implementation of control measures that reduced the opportunity for spread. While the data are too few to enable us to draw emphatic conclusions, this interpretation is supported by the finding that the number of secondary cases produced by each index case fell as the time from onset of symptoms until isolation of each case fell.

While these data suggested that SARS was only moderately infectious and could be made still less infectious through the use of rigorous control measures, the small numbers of cases meant that R_0 could not be estimated accurately from empirical data. Several different groups of epidemiologists used mathematical models to simulate the spread of SARS, arriving at an estimate of R_0 that ranged between two and four, much less than the R_0 for measles of approximately 15–20.[10, 11] While these estimates confirmed the impression that SARS was not overwhelmingly infectious, they also allowed researchers to make predictions about what might have happened had control measures not been put into place. It is important to note that even for relatively low basic reproductive numbers of 3 and 4, the vast majority of a population will ultimately become infected if nothing is done to reduce the natural transmissibility of the organism. The fact that the number of people infected by SARS was only a tiny fraction of the population suggests that control measures were highly effective and possibly prevented a much more serious pandemic.

Although the basic reproductive number of approximately three implies that there were on average only three secondary cases for each index case, the "averaging" process obscures the fact that much of the transmission that took place did so through "super-spreading" events, in which a single infectious case infected a large number of secondary cases. Many of these "super-spreading" events took place within hospitals or in unusual contexts such as the Amoy Gardens complex, where a single infected person came into contact with many other susceptibles, either directly through health-care delivery or indirectly via a faulty sewage system. Again, data from Singapore are revealing. The vast majority of infectious cases in Singapore did not go on to produce any secondary cases; most of the other infectious people infected one or two other people, while a small number of people produced a large number of secondary cases. There is no evidence to suggest that super-spreaders were infected with unusual strains of the virus or that they differed physiologically from other infected hosts. Super-spreading may represent a social rather than a physiological phenomenon, through which some individuals have the opportunity to infect more secondary cases than others.

What Needs to Be Done to Contain SARS?

The basic reproductive number can also be used as a way to assess the potential impact of control measures quantitatively. Put simply, the reproductive number of an infection needs to be brought below 1 in order to eliminate an epidemic; the closer R_0 is to 1 in the first place, the easier that task will be. In the absence of an effective vaccine or treatment for SARS, the only control measures available were the isolation of infectious people and the quarantining of people who had been exposed to infectious people but were not yet clearly infected or symptomatic. Both of these measures were put into effect in many afflicted places with varying degrees of rigor—over 30,000 people were quarantined in Beijing and many more in Hong Kong, Singapore and Taiwan. Although few doubt the wisdom of isolating people with active infection, several recent commentators have suggested that quarantining all those exposed to an infectious person may not be necessary to control SARS. The efficacy of quarantine depends on the relative infectiousness of the virus before the onset of symptoms—for diseases like chickenpox, in which people become infectious several days prior to developing the clinical disease, quarantine may prevent a substantial proportion of infections. Current data for SARS, however, suggests that infected people do not become highly infectious until well into their clinical disease, possibly as late as seven or eight days after the onset of symptoms. In this case, quarantine may not prevent many of the infections and resources would be better used to establish highly effective isolation procedures. Should SARS return in the future, it will be extremely important to estimate more precisely the timing of infectiousness relative to the onset of symptoms, because these data will help guide any future choice of public health interventions.

How Virulent Is SARS?

The "virulence" of an organism is often difficult to determine, since it reflects both the inherent capacity of a pathogen to cause disease and the vulnerability of a specific host to affliction from that disease, vulnerability that varies widely from person to person. Furthermore, a "virulent" pathogen is one that causes severe disease as well as death, and measures of disease severity are often difficult to assess. Nonetheless, virulence is often crudely quantitated by estimating the proportion of those infected who die from the disease, a measure often referred to as the "case-fatality rate." Despite the early reports from China that few of the first 300 people infected had died, the case fatality rate was found to be relatively high in comparison to other viral respiratory infections, especially among those with underlying medical conditions. Risk of death from SARS was also found to be very much determined by age; among those under age 24, fewer than 1 percent of those infected died, while risk jumped to 6 percent in those aged 25–44, 15 percent in people aged 45–64 and was higher than 50 percent in those aged 65 and older.[12] Chronic medical conditions such as underlying respiratory ailments, diabetes mellitus, heart disease, and renal failure were also strongly associated with a poor outcome, and the disease appeared to have a more severe course in pregnant women, although the infants born to infected mothers were not infected themselves at birth. Young children seemed to be remarkably unaffected by the disease, in contrast to influenza, which often afflicts the very young as well as the elderly.

Will SARS Return?

For many months after the last reported case of SARS, there has been much debate on whether SARS will return. The evidence against the return of SARS was succinctly summarized by Dr. Donald Low in a recent commentary published in a Canadian medical journal.[13] There, Low argued that SARS would be unlikely to reoccur because the infectious reservoir of the virus is limited to a few "exotic" animals sold in live-animal markets in China, laboratories in which the virus is stored under increasingly rigorous safety standards, and humans in whom symptomatic (and consequently, infectious) disease appeared to have been eradicated. Furthermore, most transmission during the epidemic occurred in hospitals, and since intensive efforts to control nosocomial spread appeared to have been effective in curtailing spread in the past, proper precautions taken in the future should limit a potential outbreak early in its course. Low concludes that the "only real threat for the reintroduction of SARS-CoV to human populations is transmission from animals in markets in the south of China," but he notes that "early recognition and institution of control measures will prevent what we witnessed in 2002–2003."

Ironically, by the time this apparently very reasonable editorial was published on January 6, 2004, the first community-acquired case of the 2004 winter season had been confirmed one day previously in Guangdong, China. So far, it is unclear how this first new case became infected, although several media reports have implicated rats found in the patient's apartment, which tested positive for SARS-CoV.

In contrast to the slow response of the Chinese government at the beginning of the 2003 epidemic, the public health reaction to this single reported case has been swift and far-reaching. Not only have eighty-one human contacts of the patient been traced and placed under observation, but the Chinese government has announced plans to slaughter civets and other animals that may pose a threat to humans. While the WHO has welcomed the decision to minimize contact between humans and the animals that may carry the virus, it has also warned that this kind of mass slaughter may pose a threat of contamination to those carrying out the work. Furthermore, if trade in exotic animals is made illegal, a black market may emerge that would be much more difficult to monitor than the existing open animal markets. Despite these practical concerns on how to implement control measures, the response from China to this recurrent threat has been clear: surveillance for SARS is being actively pursued, the process is being conducted openly, and vigorous action is being taken. Whether this change of approach will prevent an epidemic this year remains to be seen.

CHAPTER TWO

The Role of the World Health Organization in Combating SARS, Focusing on the Efforts in China

ALAN SCHNUR

The dramatic reports of an outbreak of atypical pneumonia in February 2003, affecting mainly health workers from southern China, captured the attention of the entire world. The twenty-two foreign consulates in Guangzhou informed their nationals and also their Ministries of Foreign Affairs and Health about the outbreak and disseminated information to their nationals in response to the circulating facts and rumors. There was widespread concern, and additional information was requested. The clustering of cases indicated that the new disease could be communicable, although additional information was needed to confirm this. The possibility that a lethal communicable disease spread by airborne transmission was circulating in southern China created widespread fear and panic. This fear was dramatically increased when cases of atypical pneumonia, similar to the cases being reported from Guangdong province were also reported from Vietnam and Hong Kong at the end of February and beginning of March 2003. It was then recognized that this was a new disease, with the causative agent not yet known and

Dr. Henk Bekedam, WHO Representative, and Dr. Li Ailan, Dr. Daniel Chin, Dr. James Killingsworth, and Dr. Lisa Lee, technical staff in the WHO China office at the time of the SARS outbreak, contributed to the preparation of this chapter.

without any known treatment. The name Severe Acute Respiratory Syndrome, or SARS, was given to the disease by the World Health Organization (WHO) on March 15, 2003, and actions intensified to organize an international response to it to protect global health.

The WHO is an international organization composed of 192 member states. The secretariat of the organization carries out the policies and directions laid out by the World Health Assembly, the governing body of the organization. At the time of the first SARS cases, the WHO did not have a mandate to act as an international health police to force countries to report. The WHO's role was to collect and verify official information on behalf of its member states and provide updates to the international community under the agreed international health regulations. This chapter reviews the WHO's work during the SARS epidemic, with a focus on the work done at the country level in China, which had the first reported cases and the largest number.

An Overview of the Work of the Three Levels of the WHO

The WHO normally functions at three levels: headquarters, region, and country, with the headquarters located in Geneva, Switzerland. There are six regional offices, with the Regional Office for the Western Pacific, in Manila, being the one most heavily involved in the SARS outbreak. There is a WHO country office in China, headed by the WHO representative, based in Beijing.

In general, WHO work at the headquarters level centers on normative work, policy setting, issuing of global guidelines, and global information collection, dissemination, and coordination. The regional office strongly and closely supports the country offices and also adapts the headquarters guidelines to the specific situation in the region, as necessary, and disseminates these to the countries. The country office is responsible for close interface with the government at country level, collecting and disseminating relevant health information to higher levels of the WHO and, when necessary, modifying guidelines to make them more relevant for the specific country. WHO country offices play an important role in coordinating international health work in a country, interacting with other health partners and embassies.

The International Health Regulations: Past and Future

The guiding principle for the International Health Regulations (IHR) is to prevent the spread of diseases internationally through early detection of events that threaten public health. The current IHR, first adopted in 1969, were intended to help monitor and control six infectious diseases: cholera, plague, yellow fever, smallpox, relapsing fever, and typhus.[1] The IHR were modified in 1973 and 1981 to reduce the number of notifiable diseases in line with changed conditions. The regulations provide that investigation of disease outbreaks within countries is the responsibility of each individual country. For three notifiable diseases with implications for international health: plague, cholera, and yellow fever, countries are to report cases to the WHO by the most rapid possible means. Work is currently under way to revise the IHR to bring them up to date with current disease threats and changed conditions in the twenty-first century, which makes it possible for new diseases to spread more rapidly due to globalization.

It is proposed that the revised IHR focus on syndromes as well as specific diseases, so that any new diseases can be rapidly reported. It is also proposed to cover economic and political sanctions and reactions to disease reports under the revised IHR, since they are an important component of reporting. The recent SARS epidemic once again showed the economic consequences of communicable disease reports.

The WHO's Role in Communicable Disease Reporting in China

An important component of the WHO's work in China has been to work with the Ministry of Health and other partners to establish and strengthen disease surveillance and response systems. For example, following an outbreak of Avian influenza (H5N1) in humans in Hong Kong in 1997, the WHO and the Chinese Ministry of Health organized a joint mission to Guangdong province to review the influenza surveillance system and situation in January 1998.[2] Since then, the WHO has worked with China to improve influenza surveillance.

Communicable Disease Surveillance in China

Communicable disease surveillance in China is regulated by the National Law on Communicable Diseases Prevention and Control, which when SARS first appeared had last been revised in 1989. This law mandates reporting of specified notifiable diseases and requires that each level of government receive reports of these diseases and investigate them. Reports are submitted to higher levels at fixed periods (immediately for category A diseases, as soon as possible for category B diseases, and at the end of the year for category C diseases). If one level is not able to investigate and resolve a disease report, it will request support from the next higher level.[3] Normally, counties, prefectures, and provinces try to handle disease outbreaks themselves, only calling in help if there are insufficient technical resources to diagnose and control the disease.

In the past, this system worked well, because the movement of people in China was very limited, and if help was required from higher levels, it could be requested after lower levels had first conducted a thorough investigation and implemented control measures. In this context,

SARS, which did not fall under the listed notifiable diseases, was investigated by local health officials in Guangdong, with no specific legal requirement in the initial stages to report to the central level.

SARS very clearly showed that with globalization and the greatly changed socioeconomic conditions brought about by China's economic development in the past twenty years, the current notifiable disease law is not in line with the current situation. With vastly improved communications, diseases can now spread to anywhere within China in just a few hours, as well as spread more easily from China to the rest of the world.

It was not possible to change the law during the SARS epidemic, because doing so required action by the National People's Congress, so the Ministry of Health issued a document to the provinces ordering them to report SARS cases immediately, in effect treating SARS as a category B disease. These data from the provinces were then used in the daily reports issued by the Ministry of Health (MOH).

Eventually, based on the experience with SARS, the Eleventh Standing Committee of the Tenth National People's Congress revised the 1989 National Law on Communicable Diseases Prevention and Control in August 2004, the effective date being December 1, 2004.

A Brief Chronology of Events Related to the WHO's Role in the SARS Outbreak

November 2002 to January 2003

Cases of a contagious atypical pneumonia began to spread in Guangdong province. Local and provincial health staff investigated the cases and started compiling information to allow prevention and control of the disease. The central level was informed by Guangdong province, and assistance requested, in January 2003. The WHO was only informed of the cases in February 2003, with more detailed information about the situation in Guangdong only received in March 2003.

February 2003

The Guangdong Provincial Health Bureau issued official guidelines on criteria for the diagnosis of atypical pneumonia on February 3, 2003. The guidelines provided a preliminary case definition for the cases of atypical pneumonia and recommendations on how to prevent its spread. This internal document was not provided to the WHO until April.

The WHO became involved on February 10, 2003, after receiving a telephone call from an embassy in Beijing and an email rumor about reports of a strange contagious disease in Guangdong province affecting the lungs, which had caused panic in Guangdong. The same day the WHO China office emailed the Ministry of Health requesting clarification about the rumor and the Regional Office for the Western Pacific in Manila informing them of the disease reports.[4] The WHO continued to officially request detailed information on the outbreak from the MOH throughout February and March.

There was initial concern within the WHO about influenza A (H5N1): all reports of atypical pneumonia or other illnesses that could indicate a new type of influenza are fast-tracked for concern and action. Hong Kong had reported H5N1 among chickens in December 2002, and two cases of human H5N1 infections were confirmed in Hong Kong on February 19, 2003. However, while work had to be done to exclude H5N1 influenza, WHO staff were considering the possibility of a new disease from the very first report.

Media representatives started to call and visit the WHO office in large numbers from the week of February 10 with the quantity and intensity of media interaction continually increasing until May.

The 1st WHO Mission to China (Beijing and Guangdong) with experts from the U.S. Centers for Disease Control and Prevention (CDC), Japan National Institute for Infectious Disease (NIID), WHO Western Pacific Regional Office (WPRO), and WHO China was proposed to the

MOH on February 20, 2003. Agreement was delayed by discussions on the request for the mission to also visit Guangdong province. The MOH agreed only to the Beijing visit, and the team arrived on February 23, 2003. However, detailed discussions, with details on the cases in Guangdong, only started on March 4, 2003. At the start of discussions, there was the fear that the disease could be a new influenza strain. This was based on an assumption that case reports were not complete and the higher number of reported health worker cases could reflect incomplete reporting in the community rather than a new disease. The WHO continued to push to visit Guangdong to gather data firsthand throughout the mission.

March 2003

The outbreak became global with cases reported in other countries and areas following the spread of cases at the Metropole Hotel in Hong Kong and the reporting of cases in Vietnam and Hong Kong.

The WHO issued its first global health alert on March 12, 2003,[5] describing the atypical pneumonia in Vietnam and Hong Kong. A second global alert was issued on March 15, 2003, providing the case definition, naming the new disease SARS, and providing advice to international travelers to raise awareness about the illness. This was the first global health alert issued in the history of the WHO. It provided clinical features of the disease and advised that health workers appeared to be at greatest risk. It advised that the cause of the disease was still unidentified but presumed to be an infectious agent and advised that antibiotics and antiviral drugs did not appear effective in treating it. It also advised that the disease was spreading internationally, within Asia and to Europe and North America. The case definitions for suspected and probable cases were also announced and guidelines provided for healthcare workers.[6]

The China MOH continued to maintain that atypical pneumonia in

Guangdong was not necessarily related to the SARS outbreaks in Vietnam and Hong Kong.

On March 17, 2003, the WHO established three global networks on SARS to share public information by telephone and on secure web sites, covering laboratory, epidemiology, and clinical aspects of the disease. Rapid progress was made in all three areas, but most dramatically in the laboratory network, which started unprecedented collaboration and work to rapidly identify the cause of SARS.

WHO China staff continued to hold meetings with MOH staff to brief them on international reaction, request additional information and offer support from the WHO, including a team of technical experts to visit Guangdong. A meeting was held with the minister of health on March 13, 2003.

A WHO team was finally invited to visit China to review information on the new disease, starting its work on March 24, 2003 and holding meetings with MOH and China Center for Disease Control and Prevention (CCDC) staff between March 24 and 28, 2003. During these meetings, it was agreed that the case definition for atypical pneumonia used in Guangdong province was similar to the one used for SARS and that the atypical pneumonia occurring in Guangdong province was SARS. The global case figures were subsequently updated.

While awaiting approval to visit Guangdong, the WHO team visited sites in Beijing.

April 2003

On April 2, 2003, for the first time in its history, the WHO imposed a travel advisory for Hong Kong and Guangdong, recommending that global travelers consider postponing all but essential travel to these places. This advisory was based on evidence accumulated from exported cases that three criteria were potentially important in the increasing of international spread: magnitude of outbreak and number of new cases each day, pattern of local transmission and exportation of probable cases. This information was rapidly disseminated through the WHO Internet web site. This travel advisory was made in the context of several governments having already issued travel advisories to their citizens.

A WHO team was able to visit Guangdong province from April 3 to 8, 2003. During this mission, a wealth of information and insights into the new disease became available. It was discovered that a case definition and control and treatment guidelines had been developed by Guangdong province public health staff in February, based on their investigations.[7] It was clear that the disease continued to circulate in April and had not been controlled. The differences in terminology used by Chinese officials and the international community, which resulted in a lack of trust of the officially reported figures, were pointed out by the WHO mission.

On April 6, 2003, an International Labor Organization official died of SARS in Beijing Ditan Infectious Disease Hospital. The lack of any apparent source of infection and the rapid progression from illness to death in an apparently previously healthy person shocked the international community in Beijing and greatly increased levels of concern. It was later learned that the official had been infected with SARS on a flight from Bangkok to Beijing by a person who had previously been infected on a flight from Hong Kong to Beijing.

As more was learned about the disease, it became possible to begin to identify control strategies. These were discussed during daily WHO technical teleconferences and were then recommended on the WHO web site.

The WHO mission to Guangdong presented its report to the MOH on April 9, 2003. The team advised that Guangdong was responding well to the outbreak, but that such success could not be expected if the disease should spread to other parts of China. The report was more critical of the situation in Beijing, where the work was not as well organized as in Guangdong.[8]

A work plan of provincial visits and priority activities was developed following the WHO Guangdong mission's report to the MOH on April 9, 2003. The work plan was formulated assuming that cases were occurring not only in Guangdong but in other provinces as well, given the presence of the disease during the Spring Festival, when many migrant workers returned home. There was an urgent need to improve surveillance and infection control everywhere and get reports of any suspected and probable cases. Overconfidence and complacency that existing systems of disease control and infection control could deal with the new disease were widespread, and WHO staff advised caution. It was also recommended that only specially equipped hospitals with specially trained staff should be allowed to retain and treat suspected SARS cases. The highest priority was for a WHO mission to conduct an in-depth review of the situation in Beijing.

A WHO team visited Beijing from April 11 to 15, 2003, with approval to visit any health facility, with the exception of military hospitals. However, a presentation was made by staff from one of the military hospitals, and permission was later granted for the team to visit two military hospitals on April 15, 2003. The WHO team was aware of rumors of unreported cases in government and military hospitals, with reports received from the media and also from contacts. Based on visits to several hospitals where there were rumors of unreported cases, the WHO mission concluded that there were likely probable cases of SARS that were being treated in several hospitals as "under observation" cases and thus were not reported to the MOH. The mission reported to the MOH that the current surveillance system was not adequate to detect and report all SARS cases and recommended that urgent action was needed to improve surveillance, reporting, and infection control and include all hospitals in the reporting system. The team concluded that there was the risk of an explosive outbreak in Beijing similar to those that had occurred in Guangdong and Hong Kong. The mission presented its report to the MOH on April 16, 2003.[9]

The presentation to the MOH was followed by a tumultuous question-and-answer session at the WHO office on April 16, 2003, where findings of the Beijing mission were shared with the media. Team members estimated that there might be from 100 to 200 probable SARS cases in the city, as well as over 1,000 suspected and under-observation cases. This figure contrasted sharply with the official report two days earlier of only 37 SARS cases in Beijing.

Following the removal from their posts of the minister of health, Dr. Zhang Wenkang, and the mayor of Beijing, Meng Xuenong, on April 20, 2003, it was announced that the MOH would release daily figures on new cases and those discharged from the hospital. Reporting started on April 21, 2003.

Following the mission to Beijing, a WHO team also visited Shanghai from April 21 to 26, 2003 and found that the work was going on well and there was no evidence of a SARS outbreak in the city.

In late April, the WHO brought in a travel health expert who urgently recommended that temperature screening of passengers should be started before the May Day holiday to prevent spread of the disease through transmission on planes, trains, boats, or buses.

May 2003

From a low point in the course of the epidemic in early May 2003, with more than 2,000 probable cases reported in Beijing and 100 new cases a day being reported, along with case reports from other provinces, the outbreak was gradually brought under control. Traditional basic disease-control strategies of surveillance, quarantine, isolation, and infection control proved to be adequate to stop transmission. By May 7, all probable SARS cases could be moved to specially designated hospitals, and by May 8, the epidemic in Beijing had peaked and the number of new probable cases per day had started to decline.

As part of the work plan of provincial visits, joint MOH-WHO teams visited several provinces in May: Hebei—May 8–12, Guangxi Autonomous Region—May 12–16, Henan—May 14–18, and Anhui—May 18–22, 2003.

Global health leaders attended the World Health Assembly from May 19 to 27, 2003, where SARS was one of the major topics. A resolution on SARS was passed.

On May 29, 2003, for the first time since Beijing had started reporting daily SARS cases in April, no new cases were reported. By the end of May 2003, very few SARS cases were being reported throughout China. The last cases were reported in early June.

June 2003

A high-level WHO mission visited Beijing from June 10 to 12, 2003, to review the data from all infected provinces, consider lifting the travel advisory, and revise the list of affected areas. WHO experts worked with national colleagues preparing the provincial reports to present to the high-level WHO mission, bringing essential data together for the first time.

At a joint MOH-WHO press conference in Beijing on June 12, 2003, Executive Vice Minister of Health Gao Qiang and Dr. David Heymann, WHO executive director for communicable diseases, along with Dr. Henk Bekedam, WHO China representative, announced that the work was going well. This was the first joint MOH-WHO press conference.

On June 13, 2003, the WHO announced that travel recommendations for Hebei, Inner Mongolia Autonomous Region, Shanxi, and Tianjin Municipality were being removed, and that Guangdong, Hebei, Hubei, Inner Mongolia, Jilin, Jiangsu, Shaanxi, Shanxi, and Tianjin had been removed from the list of areas with recent local transmission.

As part of the continuing work plan for provincial visits, joint MOH-WHO teams visited additional heavily affected areas: Tianjin—June 6–14, Shanxi and Inner Mongolia—June 17–25.

On June 24, at a joint press conference with the MOH, Dr. Shigeru Omi, WHO regional director for the Western Pacific, announced that

Beijing had been removed from WHO's list of affected areas and that travel recommendations were also being lifted for Beijing.

July 2003

Following control of the outbreak in Canada and Taiwan, China, the WHO announced that SARS was under control worldwide on July 5, 2003.

The WHO's Roles at Different Levels

Geneva HQ

The outbreak of a new disease presented the problem of having to learn about the disease while making policies based on the best available evidence. As Dr. Heymann said at the time, we were building the ship while sailing in it.

WHO HQ provided overall leadership and activated the Global Outbreak Alert and Response Network (GOARN), which coordinates information exchange and identifies experts to work in affected countries. Strengths and weaknesses of the GOARN system were uncovered during the SARS outbreak, because it was found that responses to the outbreak in Asia differed in several ways from previous GOARN responses, such as fighting Ebola hemorrhagic fever in least-developed countries.

WHO HQ collected and provided regular up-to-date and accurate international disease-control information to the public and the media through the global web site. Through three unprecedented global networks, scientific work was rapidly advanced to find the cause of SARS and to develop laboratory tests. Work on the epidemiology and treatment of SARS also progressed, but without the dramatic results of the laboratory network.

From early on in the outbreak, the WHO's director general and the executive director for communicable diseases in Geneva personally took part in SARS activities. Daily technical teleconferences among WHO staff and regular teleconferences of senior staff were held, where issues could be discussed and decisions taken. HQ staff offered technical and administrative support to lower levels, including offering to intervene by writing letters to governments.

The 56th World Health Assembly, the governing body of the WHO, discussed the SARS situation at its May 2003 meeting and passed a resolution endorsing the secretariat's work to date and making recommendations for further strengthening the work. Of importance in the resolution was the endorsement of the use of so-called nonofficial sources of information on communicable diseases.[10] The first information on the SARS cases in Guangdong had come from rumors and the media.

The Manila Regional Office for the Western Pacific (WPRO)

In response to the SARS threat, the WHO's Western Pacific Regional Office in Manila gave itself four principal objectives: (a) contain and control the outbreaks, (b) support the health-care infrastructure in affected countries, (c) help vulnerable countries prepare for the possible arrival of the virus, and (d) provide the latest information to health officials and address public concerns.

The regional office not only provided information, guidelines, and staff support for affected countries but also helped the countries at highest risk of becoming affected to prevent the spread of the disease. Infection-control supplies were also stockpiled in case of need. The value of these inputs were seen in Mongolia, where the guidelines proved highly effective and cases imported from China were controlled without much spread. The regional office also worked on partner and donor coordination, as well as interacting with the media.

Regional cross-border verification of reports, rumors, and patient travel was coordinated by this level. Rumors collected from many sources—national health authorities, airlines, expert teams, emails from the public, news media, the Internet, and word of mouth—were distributed to the appropriate offices for investigation and follow-up.

The following guidelines, protocols, fact sheets, and training materials were prepared by the regional office: country preparedness guidelines and checklist, national preparedness guidelines, assessment protocol for national preparedness, infection-control guidelines and tools such as a training video on infection control.

The regional office also established a procurement and logistics system for SARS infection-control equipment. As part of this work, a minimum requirement SARS kit (the WHO SARS kit) was identified and procured. With $3 million in support from the Japan International Cooperation Agency (JICA), procurement and shipping of kits to affected countries was done by the WPRO and the WHO office in Thailand

The regional director took an active part in SARS issues, including writing letters to China's minister of health to push activities and collaboration forward.

The China Country Office

Inasmuch as China was the most heavily affected country, the WHO China office quickly became fully involved in SARS control and prevention. As the workload increased, the need for additional staff became apparent. From early on in the epidemic, staff worked with the government of China to learn lessons from SARS and to strengthen the public health system to better respond to future health threats. Details of the work done by the China country office are given above.

From February 2003, a work plan for the WHO office was developed, including manpower requirements, to do the necessary work rapidly and effectively. The work plan laid out the activities to be carried out based on agreed principles and strategies. The following areas of expertise required in the office were listed in the work plan: (a) epidemiology and surveillance/response, (b) infection control, (c) laboratory aspects, (d) research, (e) travel information and recommendations, (f) media relations and information dissemination, (g) field teams for field visits, and (h) administration to service the increased number of staff and consultants. These areas could only be fully covered from mid March

2003 as staff and consultant support was provided from within the WHO and from the GOARN network. A total of more than eighty experts from fourteen countries supported WHO China office staff during the period from February to August 2003. Work was also coordinated with teams from France, Japan, and the United States, and nongovernmental organizations such as Médecins sans frontières, which supported China in SARS work. Experts were also provided directly to the WHO office by Sweden and Chile.

The WHO China office, as the center of the SARS epidemic, carried out the following activities:

—Remained in constant contact with China MOH technical and administrative staff, sending written official requests to the Department of International Cooperation of the MOH for additional information about the disease reports.

—Responded to many queries from embassies about the situation on whether it was safe to live and travel in China and whether visas could be issued to residents of Guangdong and other infected areas.

—Provided information to the media, which had started contacting the WHO, since there was a dearth of information from official sources in Guangdong and the MOH.

From February 2003 on, the WHO China office formulated and implemented the following strategies to deal with the situation:

1. Work with the MOH in the usual formal ways, but also informally with technical staff.

—Maintain confidentiality of information not officially released by the MOH, provided that withholding any confidential information would not threaten life or international public health. Given that the WHO did not have a mandate for releasing information not officially released by member states, this approach was necessary to maintain the very successful long-term working relationship with the MOH and to maintain channels for further sharing of information.

—Press the MOH for more information, such as daily reports by province, and for visits of WHO experts to the affected areas.

2. Provide updated, accurate information to all embassies and international organizations to counter the circulation of rumors. An email information update was started in February and continued to be provided regularly.

3. Assign top priority to contacts with embassies, since they report back to the Ministry of Foreign Affairs and MOH in their home countries. All phone calls from embassies were immediately answered and updated information was shared.

4. Provide information to the media on details available to the WHO in view of the dearth of information from the MOH and the CCDC.

—Media question-and-answer sessions were organized, press releases prepared and media interviews with WHO staff arranged. Often the media briefing would be held in the afternoon, after a mission had presented its report to the MOH in the morning. With tremendous interest from the media, and constant phone calls, priority was assigned to responding to the press to counteract rumors. It was feared that without reliable information, rumors like those that had caused panic in Guangzhou, and later Beijing, would prevail.

—The principle was adopted that the office would deal in a responsible manner with confidential information and that no information would be shared with the media before it was given to the MOH. Clearance was not requested from the MOH, but it was agreed that the MOH should be apprised of all recommendations, concerns, and requirements directly from the WHO and not hear about them first from the media. All WHO consultants were informed of this principle, and it was followed throughout the outbreak.

After lengthy discussions, starting in February 2003, the Chinese MOH agreed to WHO proposals for the following phases of field visits:

Phase 1: Guangdong preliminary visit and follow-up visits to go over data with local health bureau and Center for Disease Control and Prevention staff more thoroughly.

Phase 2: Beijing and Shanghai visits, with Beijing seen as the absolute top priority, given rumors of widespread cases, the presence there of embassies reporting back to their home countries, the media presence, and the potential for the spread of SARS from there to other countries and to provinces within China.

Phase 3: Visits to the highest-risk provinces—Hebei, Guangxi, Inner Mongolia, Shanxi, Tianjin, Henan—to learn about local measures and whether there had been any spread of the disease.

Phase 4: Visits to lower-priority provinces where there had been few or no cases reported, but where there was still concern that transmission could be occurring.

Discussion

As the first global health crisis of the twenty-first century, the SARS epidemic demonstrated the continuing threat posed by communicable diseases to public health and the risks of new and reemerging diseases quickly affecting all countries in the age of globalization. The WHO, as the global international health agency, played an active role in supporting countries to control the international spread of the disease and in informing the public. Shortcomings were found both at the national level in China and also at the international response level. These shortcomings need to be addressed before the next global health threat arises.

From the early days of the outbreak, the weaknesses in China's national disease-surveillance system were apparent. The shifting of funds to curative areas with the potential to generate income had caused a shortage of resources in public health areas such as disease surveillance and response. These shortcomings were to play an important role in allowing SARS to go unreported for so long and to spread so rapidly. It was mentioned by the WHO early on in discussions with the Chinese MOH that the shortage of funds for public health was adversely affecting disease surveillance and control. These issues were continually raised in meetings with senior officials in Beijing, and officials were urged to provide additional resources for public health and disease surveillance. Based on the SARS experience, the WHO China office issued a paper on public health options for China, stressing the need to strengthen preventive health services and system equity.[11]

There are many lessons to be learned from the SARS outbreak. It is impossible to completely list and discuss all of them here, but the following six key points are proposed for consideration, based on the WHO China office experience:

1. The SARS outbreak showed that communicable diseases remain a grave threat to humans and the stability of their societies. Societies are at constant risk of catastrophic spread of illness from new pathogens, particularly those spread through the respiratory route. Human society must maintain constant vigilance or face the consequences. The SARS outbreak also showed that people very much fear communicable diseases, especially respiratory diseases, where lifestyle and behavior cannot easily be modified to avoid infection. At the political level, governments need to provide leadership and funding for "public goods," particularly systems of disease surveillance and response, as a basic requirement of protecting the public and maintaining public order and prosperity. SARS in China awakened public demand for a government response to the outbreak and to improving disease surveillance and control.

2. The SARS outbreak showed the importance of international efforts to stop outbreaks of communicable disease, and that global protection against new disease threats is potentially compromised by weak disease surveillance and response systems in any country. The outbreak

confirmed the inadequacy of the current International Health Regulations to safeguard global health security. This had already been recognized, and revision was moving ahead, but the outbreak showed the importance of expediting revision of the regulations and further improving the IHR reporting and compliance requirements.

3. The weakness and vulnerability of China's public health system to sudden health emergencies due to the lack of attention paid to public goods was clearly shown. The inadequacy of China's disease reporting / response and information-exchange system was also highlighted for the entire world to see. The old model of disease surveillance and response, particularly the interaction between different levels, formulated for a very different China, clearly did not meet the requirements of the new socioeconomic conditions in the country and will need to be revised and strengthened.

4. Globalization, with its increased trade and travel, meant that outbreaks even in a small prefectural city can quickly become international in scope and threat. The lead time required to identify and deal with health threats before they become global in nature was shown to be much shorter than previously envisioned. Disease-control plans and the systems set up to monitor the potential for outbreaks of new diseases will need to be reviewed. The SARS outbreak also demonstrated the overwhelming and predominant significance of national responses to global outbreaks of disease. In the end, it was what China did that mattered most in controlling the outbreak. Reconsideration of the present public outlook that disease outbreaks are largely the problem of the country where they occur will be required. Increased consideration will need to be given to providing funding and technical support to improve national capabilities to detect and stop disease outbreaks as an essential component of safeguarding global health.

5. The timely and accurate release of information to the media must be an essential component of any public health system and disease-con-

trol effort. The importance of the media in collecting and reporting information on SARS, and their role in informing the public, as well as health experts and governments, was striking, with the outbreak again showing that rumors will fill a vacuum created by a dearth of reliable, believable information. The inadequacy of the current MOH/CCDC system for information dissemination contributed to the fear and panic, both within China and internationally, with serious economic and social consequences.

6. To control SARS, a disease for which the causative agent was not known, and for which there were no medicines to prevent or treat, the old-fashioned basic principles of disease surveillance, quarantine, isolation, and infection control were required, even in the era of molecular biology and wonder drugs. "Mass mobilization" and "mass campaigns," which had been used by China previously to fight communicable diseases, proved to be a very effective approach to combating SARS. In an era in which new diseases might arise at any time and spread rapidly, recognizing and practicing these principles will remain a very important aspect of public health work.

Will the lessons learned from the SARS outbreak be translated into action? Many things need to be done both in China and at the global level. Global information sharing and international responses need to be augmented. Funding for disease surveillance and response needs to be dramatically increased. Further research on the disease-control aspects of globalization needs to be done so that travel advisories and mass media information can be supplemented by a larger range of health-security actions and incentives. However, following control of the SARS outbreak, interest and resources appear to be declining. It remains to be seen whether the lessons learned from SARS will be fully implemented, and whether the global health community will be ready for the next disease, which may not be similar to SARS. It is not a question of "if" there will be a next time, for certainly there will be many next times, but rather of when. We shall find out how well prepared we are, and how much we have learned from the SARS outbreak, only after facing the next global epidemic.

Acknowledgments

Given the nature of the SARS outbreak, it is appropriate to include an acknowledgements section. The contribution and sacrifice of all the health workers throughout the world who selflessly risked their lives to control the outbreak and safeguard global health need to be acknowledged. In particular, the health workers who died of SARS after becoming infected during their work, including Dr. Carlo Urbani, of the WHO staff, must be recognized. We all owe them a debt of gratitude.

CHAPTER THREE

SARS and China's Health-Care Response

Better to Be Both Red and Expert!

JOAN KAUFMAN

The SARS epidemic of 2002–2003 was a wake-up call to the world about the threat of new, emerging infectious diseases. Ironically, SARS, a deadly atypical pneumonia from southern China, emerged around the same time that the Institute of Medicine of the National Academy of Sciences in Washington, D.C., issued *Microbial Threats to Health: Emergence, Detection, Response,* a report noting that "in the highly inter-connected and readily traversed 'global village' of our time, one nation's problems soon become every nation's problems."[1] The rapid global response to SARS was impressive and fortunately succeeded in averting a catastrophic pandemic. Post-9/11 investments in global health-information systems, surveillance, and rapid response alerted the world to a new epidemic at the end of 2002. Travel bans and bold action by the World Health Organization (WHO) limited the spread of SARS. International scientific collaboration helped define the virus and sequence its genome. Strategies for infection control, as well as therapeutic information were shared worldwide.[2]

Set against this impressive show of global cooperation are the events that unfolded in China from November 2002, when the outbreak began, to the summer of 2003 when, to the surprise and relief of the international community, the WHO declared China SARS-free. The Chinese government went from being a global pariah because of its initial failure to alert the world about the outbreak, which resulted in a worldwide epidemic, to being a global hero because of the disease's successful containment. Many believed in April 2003 that China's health-care system, weakened by years of underinvestment, was not up to the task. This chapter reviews China's health-care system's response to SARS and highlights its unique features that accomplished what many thought was the impossible task of bringing the SARS epidemic under control.

Background and Timeline

The SARS epidemic began in Foshan city, Guangzhou province, in November 2002 as an outbreak of atypical pneumonia.[2,3] Since animals, especially pigs and chickens, live in close proximity to humans, southern China long has been a breeding ground for new viruses. Recently, several new strains of flu have emerged from the area and moved quickly from southern China to Hong Kong with the massive movements of people across relaxed borders. Between November 16, 2002, and mid January 2003, the outbreak gained momentum in Guangdong, spread to the city of Heyang, 200 miles away, and finally reached Guangzhou, the provincial capital. During this period, misdiagnosed patients were not isolated and were transferred between hospitals, infecting other patients and health-care providers. In late January 2003, a local Center for Disease Control notified the Provincial Health Bureau, which then notified the Ministry of Health in Beijing, just as the week-long Chinese New Year holiday was beginning.[4] Pneumonia, atypical or otherwise, is not a mandatory reportable infectious disease in China and therefore did not fall under the requirements for surveillance and reporting set up for other communicable diseases,[5] allowing the initial outbreak to be kept from the public in Guangdong until February 11.[4] Moreover, the cluster of cases of this severe and deadly new pneumonia were at first mistakenly believed to be a new outbreak of avian flu virus, and the situation was further confused because of a separate cluster of deaths of confirmed avian flu during the same period in Foshan. Rumors of the "killer pneumonia" were flying in Guangzhou during the winter of 2002–3, accompanied by panic buying of white vinegar, which was believed to kill the virus, by the public. The outbreak was finally confirmed by a Guangdong Provincial Health Bureau news conference on February 11.[4]

The epidemic was reported to the WHO on February 11, 2003, only after the organization initiated an inquiry based upon reports received from Hong Kong's Global Outbreak Alert and Response Network (GOARN), and Global Public Health Intelligence Network (GPHIN). GOARN was established in 2001 (post 9/11) by the WHO to link 112 existing disease outbreak networks into an early alert system. Since its inception, GOARN has identified 538 outbreaks in 132 countries for investigation by the WHO and its partners. The GPHIN is a multilanguage, text-mining computer application developed by HealthCanada and launched in 1997. The WHO conducts keyword searches of GPHIN to locate unusual health events. Worldwide news articles and electronic discussion groups identify items for further analysis by the WHO.[2] A WHO team was dispatched from Geneva to investigate the Guangdong outbreak on February 19, but was stonewalled in Beijing. The team was not granted permission to travel to Guangdong until April 2.[3]

The failings of the Beijing authorities, either by intent or carelessness, to acknowledge and appropriately respond to the Guangzhou epidemic allowed the outbreak to spread to Hong Kong, and from there to elsewhere in the world. An infected doctor who had cared for SARS patients in a Guangzhou hospital flew to Hong Kong on February 21 to attend a wedding and transmitted the virus to numerous guests at the Metropole Hotel. These guests set off a serious epidemic in Hong Kong, and some of them further dispersed the virus when they flew to their homes in Singapore, Toronto, and Vietnam. Epidemics began in those places as well, and on March 12, for the first time in its history, the

WHO issued a global health alert, strengthened on March 15, and recommended against travel to all affected countries.[3]

Meanwhile, the Beijing epidemic gained momentum as infected travelers to Guangzhou infected co-passengers on airplanes and health workers in Beijing's military hospitals. Beijing authorities downplayed the extent of the epidemic in the capital, going so far as to conceal patients from visiting WHO teams.[6] A full analysis of the politics of SARS and the failures of governance associated with China's early response to the epidemic are described elsewhere in this volume.[7] Important to note, however, is that these failures in early acknowledgement and appropriate response in the capital during March and April set the stage for China's massive SARS epidemic in the following months.

In early April, as rumors in Beijing increased about unreported SARS cases in military hospitals, the Ministry of Health reported to China's State Council that "SARS was effectively under control," and that there were only 12 cases in all in the capital. By April 9, the official number of SARS cases had increased to only 22, with four deaths. Finally, however, an outraged doctor from a Beijing military hospital reported to the media that there were over 120 cases at the Number 301 PLA hospital and two other military hospitals in Beijing.[9]

In a move that surprised the world, the Chinese government fired the minister of health, Zhang Wenkang, and the deputy mayor of Beijing, Meng Xuenong, on April 20. The government dramatically changed course, instituting a rarely seen transparency and honesty in reporting, and allocating two billion yuan in emergency funding for national SARS control. Following the April 20 sacking of Zhang and Meng, the government revised the capital's SARS case number to 339, ten times that reported one week earlier. Despite the firing of senior officials and the government's admission of the full extent of Beijing's SARS epidemic, public panic resulted. With millions of economic migrants fleeing the city out of fear of being detained and quarantined, Beijing's west railway station was packed. Migrants have a history of maltreatment at the hands of Beijing police, and their civil rights are usually ignored in times of crisis for reasons of political expediency. During this period, everyone from the WHO representative in Beijing to Premier Wen Jiabao expressed deep concern that SARS might spread to the countryside, where China's rural health system had "collapsed." Worldwide focus shifted to whether China's rural health system would be able to handle large numbers of SARS cases. As cases appeared outside of Beijing and Guangdong, in Inner Mongolia, Tianjin, Shanxi, Hubei, and twenty-five other provinces, these worries increased. By May 20, there were 5,248 cases of SARS in China.[10] Toward the end of the worldwide epidemic (August 7, 2003), of the total 8,422 cases and 916 deaths in thirty countries and Hong Kong, 5,327 and 349 deaths were in China, or a full 63 percent of all SARS cases worldwide.[10]

China's Health-Care System: Twenty Years of Deterioration in Public Health Preparedness

Concerns about China's health-care system are well-founded. The past twenty years have witnessed the dismantling of China's socialist rural medical care system and its transformation into a privatized one, where poverty is closely associated with poor care and lack of access to care, and medical expenses have become a major cause of falling into poverty.[11] In 1978, China's rural, community-based primary health-care system was extolled as a model for the world at the WHO's Alma Ata conference, where the slogan "Health for all by the year 2000" was adopted.[12] By the year 2000, in its yearly World Health Report, the same organization ranked China number 188 out of 191 countries in terms of fairness in financial contribution to health.[13] In a survey conducted in 2001, 21.6 percent of rural households had fallen below the poverty line due to their medical expenses. The average cost of hospitalization is equal to an entire year of the average rural family's income (1,500 yuan, or about $175).[14] Rural Chinese seek health care based upon what they can afford, and care is often provided by traditional or minimally trained and supervised rural doctors in local clinics with poor infection-control practices.

While few would glorify the sophistication and quality of China's rural medical care system in the 1970s, many long for a return to its equity and emphasis on prevention. The care, while basic, was available to all at little cost and was combined with health education and public investments in a healthy environment. By the end of the 1970s, over 90 percent of rural citizens were covered by a medical insurance system.[14] The cooperative medical system (CMS), was based upon a referral system that began at the community level and was supported by increasingly sophisticated medical care at township and county levels. The community level curative health system of basic care provided by minimally trained health workers ("barefoot doctors") was supported by investments in preventive health care through "patriotic health campaigns" consisting of public works (like mosquito control and clean water projects) and educating the public about the prevention of disease (hand-washing, prenatal care, etc.).

After the breakup of the commune system in the late 1970s, the rural CMS was dismantled, and health-care financing was delegated to provinces and local areas, which turned to the market economy to provide the necessary money. As public finances decreased, the unregulated market (especially for drugs) steadily increased the price of care. Limited public finances were diverted to cover staff salaries at county- and township-level facilities and for other recurrent costs. Rural citizens who could afford to do so bypassed expensive township facilities for county-level care, undermining the three-tiered referral chain and distorting the value of manpower investments and training in rural health care. By 1992, only 10 percent of rural residents were still covered by rural health insurance.[14] The current system, with its focus on fee-based financing of curative care, has shifted attention and investments away from vital public health education and public works that prevent both chronic and infectious diseases. In fact, the level of curative care in rural China has greatly improved by contrast with earlier years. Most essential drugs are available in the most remote parts of the country, and staff are trained in their use; but the cost of care and the breakdown in the government's preventive public health functions have created serious inequities and distortions in the rural health system.

Of particular concern for a SARS response, the training of rural health workers is weakly financed, and standard infection-control procedures are hardly standard practice outside urban hospitals, as evidenced by high rates of hepatitis B and other blood-borne infections transmitted by improperly sterilized needles. Key public health responsibilities like surveillance and health education have been weakened over the past twenty years. Economic development goals have taken precedence over investments in public health. Poor communities invest their limited local resources to build roads to the county town or city rather than in maintaining public health systems.

Recently, rural health-care weaknesses have received attention from the national government. In 2001, "Guidance for Reforming and Developing Rural Health" was issued.[15] Jointly developed by the State Council's System Reform Office, the Ministries of Health, Agriculture, Finance, and the State Planning Commission, this document signaled the government's intention to invest heavily in rural health reform. In 2002, the central government convened a national conference to tackle issues of public financing for rural health care, the breakdown of public health systems, and maintaining quality and standards of care. The document and conference produced specific plans to rebuild infrastructures, improve surveillance of infectious diseases, revitalize maternal and child health, increase public health education and health personnel training, institute an affordable and equitable rural health insurance system, and devise a mechanism for medical financial aid to poor families.

However, twenty years of fiscal and political devolution have also made the provincial governments increasingly independent of Beijing.

Thus national-level solutions to the rural health system crisis, no matter how well intended, will be hard to carry out. China's national ministries may set policy and program guidelines, but real control over decisions and budgets rests with provincial and local governments. The Health Ministry is an especially weak player on the national, provincial, and local levels, where political and economic priorities are of greater perceived importance than public health. This has been evident in China's response to its escalating AIDS epidemic. Officials in Henan province, one of the AIDS epicenters, have blocked accurate reporting, research and prevention efforts. Despite pressure from Beijing, Henan officials have engaged in a cover-up for years and remained in their jobs.[16]

Guangdong authorities may also have concealed the gravity of the early SARS epidemic. Anxious to avoid criticism for their mishandling of earlier outbreaks, and in an effort to maintain Guangdong as the hotbed of Chinese business dynamism and economic growth, they minimized the situation. Yet barely anyone attended the annual Canton Trade Fair because of concern about SARS. Only when SARS became a political issue, an embarrassment for Beijing, did the central government impose its authority on Guangdong.

The international loss of face and China's dramatic policy reversal after April 20, 2003, set in motion the actions that brought SARS under control. What happened next is a global lesson in how political will and national mobilization are required for tackling serious threats to public health and provides important lessons for China's long-overdue response to its growing epidemics of AIDS, tuberculosis, and hepatitis. China's extensive health infrastructure, albeit weakened by years of underinvestment, rose to the occasion once national leadership provided the mandate for action. Few countries in the world have China's capacity for national mobilization, which extends to the remotest corners of this large and increasingly decentralized nation.

China's National SARS Response: Mass Mobilization for Prevention

Once the government acknowledged the full extent of the Beijing epidemic in late April, it instituted preventive measures to minimize the spread of SARS within the capital and beyond. These measures were aimed at early identification and isolation of cases and reducing public crowding and the opportunities for transmission. A national SARS headquarters was set up in Beijing under the direction of Wu Yi, acting minister of health and a vice premier. SARS was finally classified as an infectious disease, subject to the reporting requirements specified under the Law on Prevention and Control of Contagious Disease,[5] and additional legislation in the form of regulations dealing with SARS prevention and control was enacted, which required daily reporting and control measures. After April 20, daily reports of new or suspected SARS cases and deaths were required from all provinces and were reported to the WHO. The government announced free treatment for all cases of SARS as a way to encourage poorer citizens to seek care promptly.

In the early stages of the Beijing epidemic, SARS patients were hospitalized in infectious disease wards or transferred to the main infectious disease hospitals in Beijing, the Ditan and You'an hospitals. After many health-care providers fell ill due to inadequate infection control measures, a SARS hospital, Xiaotangshan, was constructed in a rural county outside Beijing. National infection-control guidelines for health-care workers were developed and proper medical waste disposal was instituted. In Beijing, suspected and confirmed SARS patients were quarantined. Sometimes all those who worked or lived in the same building were required to quarantine themselves for twelve days even if they did not have direct contact with the suspected case. This approach met with much criticism and did not conform to WHO quarantine guidelines, whereby only those directly exposed to a confirmed or suspected case of SARS are isolated. Fears of quarantine and the possibility of being sent to a SARS facility, where exposure to patients who were actually infected was likely, were major factors contributing to the exodus of Beijing residents in the early stages of the epidemic.

The Beijing government also instituted morning fever checks for all students and established fever clinics to isolate and observe febrile persons, students and otherwise. Beijing cancelled most public gatherings and closed elementary schools. The national government cancelled the annual week-long May Day holiday to minimize travel to and from Beijing, and instituted fever checks for travelers at major transportation points such as airports and bus and train stations.[17] Beijing instituted routine disinfection of public places, including taxis and buses. Finally, stricter control of live animal markets in southern China, where the virus likely originated, was imposed. Despite recent articles suggesting that some controls may be loosened, there appears to be a genuine effort to monitor emerging infectious diseases from these markets more closely.

A Case Study of SARS Control in One Poor Rural County

Despite the dismal state of the rural health system and the increasing independence of China's thirty provinces, the country controlled the spread of SARS to rural areas. High-level political accountability for the spread of SARS and national funding helped limit the epidemic. Local leaders applied impressive organizational skills to protect the public's health by quickly identifying and isolating cases, using provincial government and Beijing funding. Such a national mobilization for public health had not been seen in decades.

The story of how one poor rural county in China's south organized itself to deal with the SARS threat provides a window into the local actions that collectively contributed to national success. This county is the home to 80,000 migrants, many of whom work in Beijing and fled back to their homes in April and May. I visited it in the summer of 2003 and learned about the local response to SARS. Up to the time of my visit, the county had had no SARS cases. Two migrants had been isolated as suspected cases but were later found to have other illnesses.

This county, a designated poor county in one of China's southern provinces, is typical of many in rural China. Among the population of 900,000 rural citizens, 80,000 have abandoned farming and become economic migrants to China's booming cities, mainly Guangzhou and Beijing. Their remittances home have increased their families' household wealth, providing the impetus for more migration. Like many other counties in China's rural hinterland, they have been left behind in the country's booming economy. The annual per capita county income ranges from 977 to 1,389 yuan, or from U.S.$130 to $170. Geographically isolated, the county government has allocated the funds available to it to road construction and other infrastructure that has a direct impact on its economic development. There has been little investment in health over the past twenty years. The limited funds earmarked for health are used entirely to cover county and township salaries (supplying only 60 percent of the amount necessary; fees have to make up the remaining 40 percent). Recent rural health financing improvements are the direct result of participation in an international donor-financed project in thirty-seven poor counties nationwide.

Prior to April 20, 2003, the county leadership seemed barely aware of the SARS threat. After the health minister and Beijing deputy mayor were fired, the province and county prepared for the potential threat. With funds provided by the provincial government and donations from a national political party (a 100,000-yuan contribution given as part of an existing work unit–"sister" relationship), an existing building on the town's outskirts was converted into a SARS hospital and opened in June. (Prior to June, the county hospital had had a designated SARS ward). This local "Xiaotangshan," named after Beijing's suburban SARS hospital, was staffed by twenty-two temporarily reassigned county health workers (from the county hospital, maternal and child health hospital, etc.). These workers were trained for one week by the provincial health bureau and further trained by the district and county health bureaus in SARS prevention, clinical care, infection control, surveillance, and reporting requirements. Medical staff were housed in a separate building close to the hospital. The hospital itself had three fully separated sections: five rooms with individual beds for quarantined patients, five rooms with individual beds for suspected cases, and twenty rooms with single beds for definite SARS cases on a separate floor of the building. On the walls of the main hall of the staff building were fifteen sets of regulations concerning SARS, most produced by the provincial health bureau, dealing with reporting requirements, waste disposal, protocols for isolation and treatment of cases, quarantine procedures, prevention, and so on. Medical equipment, including respirators, was temporarily moved to the SARS hospital from other facilities in the county.

Before the SARS epidemic, the county administration did not know how many migrants there were in the county. But one of the first actions after April 20 was to conduct a complete county census to identify numbers of, and households with, migrant workers. The county now has information on all of its 80,000 migrants. In one township I visited, there were 1,700 migrants out of a population of 28,000, or about 6 percent of the population, half of whom were women. Village residents throughout the county were aware of the SARS problem. Nearly every household in this county (over 90 percent), and in most of rural China, has a television set, and after April 20, the public heard constant calls for vigilance to prevent further spread of the SARS virus. Villagers were also locally instructed to report any returning migrants to village and township authorities. Migrants returning from an infected area were required to quarantine themselves at home for twelve days. Health workers from township hospitals and health centers were dispatched to monitor the temperatures of all returned migrants on a daily basis. The health worker was required to notify the township health bureau of any febrile persons. The township would then dispatch a team to transfer the individual to Xiaotangshan for an additional twelve days of observation and quarantine. Two suspected cases were identified and transferred in this manner but did not have SARS.

During a visit to a health clinic at the level of an "administrative village" (a grouping of about ten natural villages), staffed by a former barefoot doctor who had been practicing there for over twenty years, I tried to ascertain the level of preparedness to receive a potentially SARS-infected patient. This type of clinic is the most typical first "port of call" for a villager sick with flu. There were a large number of prescription drugs available at the clinic, and the doctor was very knowledgeable about their proper use. The sale of these drugs contributes a substantial part of her income. The doctor, a woman in her fifties, readily admitted that she was unprepared, but also noted that the township had set up a system (described above) whereby no one who suspected they might have SARS would come to this clinic. Instead, they would be identified at their homes by township health workers and transferred to Xiaotangshan. She had, however, sold her entire supply of *banlangen*, the traditional Chinese medicine used for "cooling," which is believed to boost the immune system and prevent SARS if taken daily. She had to pay double the price from her supplier for the medicine during this period and thus sold it for a higher price. She also noted that it had been difficult to buy white vinegar in the county, as vinegar is also believed to prevent SARS.

This county's approach to SARS control was duplicated in almost all of China's 3,000 rural counties. SARS control became a political issue as well as a health issue, and because local officials believed their political careers were on the line, they devoted resources, their organizational skills, and their authority to instituting effective measures. Although this rural county did not have a single case of SARS, it will be better prepared in the future to identify and isolate SARS cases rapidly.

There are many lessons to be learned from China's SARS epidemic, for both China and the world. For China, the SARS epidemic was a painful lesson that integration with the global economy that has fueled China's recent unparalleled economic growth also requires better global citizenship. For the world, easy, large-scale air travel for both business and tourism can also be a rapid conduit for spreading what were once local and isolated disease outbreaks. Since infectious diseases do not respect international borders, China must do a better job of surveillance and honest, early admission and reporting of emerging infectious diseases. In fact, post-SARS China has been cooperating with the WHO to improve disease surveillance and reporting.[17, 18] The SARS epidemic was also a wake-up call for China's government on the deterioration of the public health capacity and equity of China's rural health system. Twenty years of privatization have created a distorted and inequitable rural health system. Without the political mobilization and financing put in place for SARS prevention, it is unlikely the rural health system would have been able to deal with the burden of SARS care.

Fortunately for the world, the major weapon for SARS prevention did not require sophisticated technology or complicated clinical protocols, neither of which China's rural health system could have mustered. Nineteenth-century infection-control measures for identification, isolation, quarantine, and disinfection were the means used to break the person-to-person chain of disease transmission. In China, where individual civil liberties are rarely prioritized over issues of public safety or order, the government apparatus was able to detain and isolate citizens even when they had had no direct exposure to a confirmed SARS patient. In fact, it was this fear of being unreasonably quarantined that led migrants to flee Beijing in late April. Here, also, China was able to fall back on traditions of public health mobilization from the 1960s and

1970s. This mobilization was precisely what was required to put in place the series of preventive measures that broke the chain of transmission.

Another SARS lesson was the recognition of the crucial role the media can play in calming public fears by providing accurate information. For a short while, the media were allowed to honestly report about SARS and the massive government efforts to control the epidemic, thus helping the government regain control over public information about the disease. Prior to April 20, rumors spread by mobile phone text messages and the Internet were the main sources of public information. This contributed to public panic and anger with the government. Even in China, information control is impossible in the electronic age. The role of the media must, therefore, be seen in relation to other sources of public information; and misinformation or concealment will be judged harshly. China's leaders appear to have recognized that they were quickly losing the SARS battle in the court of public opinion, and in response media controls were loosened, at least temporarily.

Finally, many hope that China's experience with SARS will be translated into a more transparent and open response to China's mounting AIDS epidemic. The same issues of transparency, media control, concealment, government leadership, and the accountability of public officials can all be applied to the way China has dealt with its AIDS epidemic over the past decade. AIDS is spread less easily than SARS, and its slow progression from infection to illness makes it less immediately frightening. However, the stigma and embarrassment associated with its two main routes of transmission, sex and drugs, makes AIDS much harder to openly discuss and address. Nonetheless, there is no question that if it is not controlled, AIDS will have a serious economic and social impact in China, as tragically evidenced by several sub-Saharan African countries. Unlike SARS, the government has not held officials responsible or accountable for transparency and action in AIDS control. National political leadership and financing have not occurred (two billion yuan was devoted to the SARS battle, but only 100 million yuan has been allocated for all national AIDS-prevention effort at the time this chapter was written—it was substantially increased in 2004). AIDS surveillance has been inadequate, making it nearly impossible to understand the full extent of the epidemic in the general population. Furthermore, China's weakened rural health system is finding it hard to handle the increasing burden of AIDS patients without the necessary resources, training, and medicines. China's response to SARS succeeded because of an infusion of financing and political will from Beijing, which focused local officials on the public health emergency. These lessons should be extended to China's battle against AIDS before it is too late.

PART II

Economic and Political Consequences

CHAPTER FOUR

Is SARS China's Chernobyl or Much Ado About Nothing?

TONY SAICH

The outbreak of severe acute respiratory syndrome, or SARS, was the first serious test faced by China's new leaders, President and General Secretary Hu Jintao and Premier Wen Jiabao, after the leadership transfer in March 2003. Before they could develop an effective profile of their own, they were knocked off course, but SARS may have provided them with an unprecedented opportunity to establish themselves as modern leaders concerned for the welfare of their people. It probably never occurred to Hu and Wen as they surveyed the policy minefields ahead that their first test would come from the health sector. It is even more unlikely that they realized that it would be a health problem with international consequences that would cause the party's credibility to be called into question.

A number of writers have speculated on the consequences of SARS for China's political evolution and opinions have ranged from the very optimistic—that it would usher in significant systemic change—to those who envisage next to no long-term impact. The specter of a "Chernobyl factor" that would produce dramatic systemic change in fact seems a remote possibility, and "old politics" began to reassert itself after Hu and Wen won their "war on SARS."[1] The different factions in the party began to jockey to take credit for the "victory," while the party as a whole began to extol its triumph in taming the viral beast. The traditional propaganda system soon found its footing to portray the struggle in terms of patriotism and turned out little ditties such as "Angels in White Coats" that pay homage to the nurses and doctors of China who, moved by love of the party and concern for the people, have worked tirelessly. Normality even returned in relations with Taiwan. Having allowed a delegation from the World Health Organization to go to Taiwan for humanitarian reasons, China made sure that this would not lead to Taiwan gaining WHO observer status and, as usual, killed such a proposal in the committee stage.

This seems to suggest that the effects of SARS on the political system are minimal at best. This may underestimate the impact over the longer term. The final impact and outcome depends on whether the virus returns in winter and spring of 2003–4 and how the government deals with it should this occur. However, Hu and Wen's approach from mid April on greatly enhanced their standing and will allow them to use SARS to push forward their own political agenda. Unlike Jiang Zemin (the former general secretary) and his supporters, who looked irrelevant and out of touch, they appeared businesslike, open, and willing to adopt modern management techniques. This should consolidate their position within elite politics. With the outbreak contained, Hu and Wen can concentrate on promoting social development to accompany economic growth, enhancing accountability within bureaucratic ranks, and restructuring the media to serve better the long-term objectives of the Chinese Communist Party (CCP). They will also need to address the urban elite's lack of trust in party "infallibility," which the cover-up and tardy response heightened.

This chapter looks first at why it took the Chinese political system so long to react to SARS, thus inducing a crisis that may have been unnecessary. Second, it looks at five areas where lessons need to be learned and how the Chinese leadership has responded. By way of conclusion, it looks at how the policy response to SARS may help the policy agenda of the new leadership.

The Politics of SARS: New Disease, New Leaders, Old System

One of the most pressing questions to be resolved is why it took from November until mid April for the Chinese leadership to take decisive action. In part, this entails trying to understand who knew what and when. A number of factors, both systemic and specific, contributed to the situation. The fact that China was undergoing a major leadership transition that started formally in November 2002 at the Sixteenth Party Congress and only ended in March 2003 with the Tenth National People's Congress meant that leaders were not only preoccupied with political jockeying, but also no one wanted to be the bearer of bad tidings. Second, leadership obsession with social stability and economic development meant that there was no incentive to release information about the disease for fear that it might cause panic or might slow down economic growth through reduced consumption or investor flight.[2] Third, there were strong bureaucratic disincentives. The Ministry of Health (MOH) is a weak player institutionally and is subordinate to party organs at the local levels. Thus, if local party leaders receive and transmit messages to downplay the disease, there is little that health officials can do. In addition, there is a lack of clarity about who to report to and under what circumstances. In accordance with Chinese law, epidemics fall under the classification of state secrets and the localities do not have the power to make public comments about disease outbreaks before this has been announced by the authorities at the national level. There is no incentive for local officials to report bad news before they have a clear signal to do so. This encourages optimistic reporting and the suppression of bad news. As discussed below, the interplay of these factors led to a delay in timely reporting and exacerbated the impact of the disease, causing precisely the kind of domestic and international crisis that the system is designed to prevent.

A Local Affair?

It is not easy to identify a new virus, and this must be especially difficult in South China, where SARS originated.[3] The area has been the point of origin for a number of flu outbreaks, and eating habits and the close proximity of livestock to humans make it ripe for producing new strains of disease. Thus, with presumably mutating strains occurring each year, how do local health officials decide what is important and what might become a dangerous new viral strain? In this context, it is interesting to note that the World Health Organization (WHO) congratulated the local health authorities on identifying the new virus rather quickly. Indeed, a researcher (Dr. Zhang Nanshan) from the Guangzhou Institute of Respiratory Disease rejected the idea that "human delay" had been involved. He pointed out that while the first case had been detected in December, it took some time for the scale of the infections to become apparent before it broke out on a large scale in Guangzhou. According to this account, once Guangdong had ascertained its seriousness at the end of January, the local authorities promptly reported this to the MOH and the central authorities.[4] This contains elements of truth, but politics did intervene to ensure that knowledge was not shared widely enough.

The first known patient actually caught the disease on November 16, 2002, in Foshan, around the time that the new party leadership was settling itself into Guangdong.[5] The new party secretary was Zhang Dejiang (formerly Zhejiang party secretary), regarded as a close supporter of Jiang Zemin, who promoted the latter's thesis that social stability and economic growth are of paramount importance, as well as Jiang's "Three Represents" platform.[6] This was not a predisposition that lent itself to thinking about social issues and public welfare.

It seems certain that Guangdong authorities knew about the disease by early January at the latest. From December 15 on, the number of patients with a form of atypical pneumonia had been increasing in

Heyuan City (about 100 miles northeast of Guangzhou). The provincial center for disease control sent a team to investigate and on January 3, they sent a fax to calm the local population, which was published in the next day's edition of the *Heyuan News*.[7] This produced a brief flurry of reporting before the Guangdong authorities stepped in to prevent any further coverage. It seems that the main motivation for stopping any further reporting was to ensure that the Chinese New Year holiday at the end of January would not be disrupted and that citizens would continue to spend.[8] However, the limited press coverage that was allowed was designed to ridicule the idea that there was anything untoward happening. The articles followed government claims that "there is no epidemic" and that the idea that there was an identified virus on the loose was "rumor." The explanation given was that the illness was the "result of changes in the weather leading to a decline in people's immune systems."[9]

Publicly, there was silence until February 11, when after outbreaks in Zhongshan and Guangzhou, a press conference was convened to still public concern. The provincial health authorities had informed doctors in Guangzhou that something was afoot and that they should isolate patients and wear masks, but the information was not made public.[10] On February 3, the Guangdong health department issued a notice on "preventing and treating the unclear pneumonia" and demanded that the illness be managed temporarily as a B-type infectious disease.[11] By early February, although Dr. Zhang mentions late January, the authorities in Beijing were being made aware of the situation in Guangdong. The Guangdong party committee and the provincial government filed a report to the MOH on February 7, and on February 9, the ministry sent Vice-Minister Ma Xiaowei with a team to investigate the situation. Thus officials in the State Council certainly knew about the situation by this time, if not before. In fact, the Guangdong party secretary, Zhang Dejiang, was a member of the Politburo and thus had ample opportunity to bring the matter to the attention of China's highest leadership had he considered it important enough. There are claims that the February 7 provincial report was read by members of the Standing Committee of the Politburo.[12]

Citizen concern expressed through the rapidly expanding new technology of instant messaging forced the Guangdong leadership to make some kind of public acknowledgement. Again, the response was to acknowledge that while there may have been a problem, it was not serious and there was no longer anything to worry about. It is not known whether sympathetic people leaked the contents of the report, but according to Guangdong Mobile, the message "There is a fatal flu in Guangzhou" was sent 40 million times on February 8, 41 million times the next day, and 45 million times on February 10.[13] With party control over information systems breaking down, there had to be a response.

On February 11, Party Secretary Zhang asked health officials to hold a press conference to put a stop to the unofficial communications that were taking place. That same day, the *Guangzhou Daily* ran a story that the virus had infected over 300 people and that 5 had died. There are claims that the paper had evaded the party secretary's ban on reporting by seeking permission from the provincial governor, Huang Huahua.[14] If true, there are overtones of factional struggle in this, because the party secretary, Zhang, was a protégé of Jiang Zemin's, whereas the governor is thought to be close to Hu Jintao. The press conference officially announced the disease for the first time but again sought to dispel any public panic by stating clearly that it was under control. This was a regular pattern to be repeated until April 20. Each time the authorities were compelled to release information, they claimed that everything was under control. The fact that the number of infections jumped from just over 300 to nearly 800 by the end of the month, with 31 deaths, would suggest otherwise. However, it seems that the panic buying in Guangzhou and elsewhere had alerted the Ministry of Public Security and it had told local officials to concentrate on social stability at the time of the press conference.

When journalists asked a local health official, Huang Qingdao, why the outbreak had not been reported earlier, he replied that "atypical pneumonia is not a disease we're legally required to report, so we didn't feel it was necessary to make it public. Now because it has had a big social impact, we decided to make it public."[15] This is a point worth considering, because it helps explain the predicament of local officials should they wish to take action on new diseases. Not surprisingly, the legal background is confusing, and different laws contradict one another. The 1988 State Secrets Law is supplemented by a 1996 set of implementing regulations concerning health-related issues.[16] The 1989 Law on the Prevention and Treatment of Epidemics is also important. According to the 1996 implementing regulations, SARS would have fallen under the category of highest-level secret (*jia lei*), since it was a widespread infectious disease, like viral hepatitis.[17] As a result, it could not be disclosed until the MOH or those organs authorized by the ministry had made the disclosure. This would mean that without ministry disclosure any local official talking publicly about the disease would be liable for prosecution. This is a disincentive for transparency, to say the least.

This problem was picked up in a May 13 *China Daily* article. The article referred to the 1989 law on treatment and prevention of epidemics and pointed out that although SARS had reached national proportions by March, it was still the local levels that were dealing with the disease. This created a problem, because only the State Council and the MOH were empowered to classify a new contagious disease. This restricted the capacity of the local levels, since they could only use the law as a reference point and could not undertake the necessary policy measures. Because the disease appeared to be limited to Guangdong (one administrative jurisdiction), this did not trigger a national response, with disastrous consequences. It was not until April 8 when it was long clear that this was no longer a "local" phenomenon that the MOH listed SARS as a statutory epidemic.

Following the press conference, despite attempts to play things down, there was more reporting, but still it was a month before more figures were published officially. Party Secretary Zhang tried to keep a lid on things and on February 14 ordered provincial authorities to educate the public to "voluntarily uphold social stability, not believe in rumors, not spread rumors" and to focus on the objective of the Sixteenth Party Congress to build China into a moderately well-off society (*xiaokang shehui*). The *Southern Daily* claimed that police had ordered operators of leading web sites to carry only positive reports on the handling of the disease.[18]

A National and Global Problem

Thus bureaucratic and other factors delayed Guangdong's response, and similar factors also affected Beijing's. While it is clear that central leaders must have known about the disease in February, the initial response was very slow. In part, this may have been because of underestimation of its impact and the belief that it was localized in the south. However, even as more information became available, no senior official would have been in much of a position to undertake action, because they were preparing for the National People's Congress that was due to open on March 5. As normal, reporting was even more tightly controlled than usual at the time of the Congress, and the media were required to present only positive news and concentrate on the events at the Congress itself. This was even more the case in 2003, because the Congress was to mark the final stage of the formal leadership transition from Jiang Zemin to Hu Jintao. Thus, on March 9, officials from the MOH met with the heads of major Beijing hospitals to inform them about SARS but told them that this was not for public distribution and certainly should not be repeated to the media.[19]

This period of delay for the Congress was fatal in terms of preventing the spread of the disease in the Chinese capital. At the Congress, a group of thirty delegates from Guangdong did table a motion calling for the establishment of a nationwide epidemic prevention network, but it was not acted upon. This may have been a way for delegates to try to register their concern. However, forces had been set in motion that would put the Chinese leadership under sufficient pressure to shift their position and to begin to deal with the SARS epidemic.

On March 15, three days before the NPC concluded its meeting, the World Health Organization (WHO) issued its first global warning about SARS, but the Propaganda Department instructed the Chinese media not to report it.[20] After the Congress, things began to change, but it took international pressure and domestic dissent to force China's leaders to take action. It is unlikely that without the pressure from international organizations such as the WHO and the postponement or cancellation of high-profile events such as the World Economic Forum China Business Summit and a Rolling Stones concert, the leadership would have changed their approach of assuring in public that all was under control, while seeking internally to block the spread of the virus.

On March 26, the authorities admitted that SARS was being dealt with in Beijing hospitals, but the news was restricted to a small mention on inside pages of newspapers and contained the upbeat view that "imported atypical pneumonia in our city has been effectively controlled."[21] On March 28, China finally informed the WHO that it would classify SARS as a category B disease, meaning that from now on provincial authorities were obliged to notify central authorities of any cases. Experts from the WHO had arrived in Beijing on March 23, and on April 2, the WHO issued an advisory warning people against travel to Guangdong and Hong Kong. The impact of SARS was becoming hard to ignore, yet it would still take Hu Jintao and Wen Jiabao another two weeks before they could lay the groundwork for a dramatic shift in policy.

On April 2, Wen Jiabao presided over a meeting of the State Council Executive Committee that heard a report from the MOH that told them that SARS had "already been brought under control."[22] This misleading report may explain why Minister Zhang Wenkang was eventually dismissed, because it subsequently became clear that the disease was far from under control. The meeting also set up a small leadership group under Zhang to oversee the work of SARS control and to coordinate with the WHO. Some report that Beijing municipal authorities and the MOH were aware of the problem but suppressed the information and thought they could deal with it. For example, on March 27, a leading Beijing virologist warned senior MOH officials and was told that they were aware of the problem but could not act, since they had to negotiate with other government departments.[23]

In this new position, Minister Zhang held a press conference on April 3 that repeated the notion that all was under control and that the number of cases in Beijing was very small: only twelve, with three deaths. This was enough for a retired army doctor, Jiang Yanyong, who knew that in one Beijing military hospital alone (no. 309) there were sixty patients and seven had died. His ire and that of his colleagues at the cover-up led him to fax CCTV and Phoenix TV from Hong Kong with his complaint. The information was ignored but given to *Der Spiegel* and *Time* magazine who put it on their web sites, leading to a deluge of critical articles in the foreign press that were read by educated urban Chinese or were translated into Chinese and circulated.[24] In light of these information flows, it was becoming increasingly difficult for the Chinese authorities to maintain the stance that there was a small problem but that basically everything was under control.

On April 4, at Wen's behest, Vice-Premier Wu Yi visited the Chinese Center for Disease Control, where she delivered a strong message that health work was very important and that "top priority" should be given to controlling SARS and implementing preventive measures.[25] As a result the director of the center, Li Liming, apologized to a press conference that excluded foreigners, stating that China's "medical departments and the mass media" had suffered from poor coordination.[26] However, the mainland media did not print the apology.

Things began to unfold more rapidly. On April 7, Premier Wen himself visited the center, and while the public reporting was positive, it seems that he criticized the military for not reporting on SARS cases and called on people to start telling the truth.[27] On April 13, at a national meeting on SARS prevention, Wen said that although the situation was "under effective control," it remained "extremely grave." Rather than being a nuisance in the way of economic progress, he announced that SARS "directly affects the overall situation of reform, development and stability" and called for better cooperation between the various departments.[28] The latter could also be taken as a criticism of the military system and its reluctance to divulge statistics to the civilian authorities. On April 13, while Hu Jintao was still visiting Guangdong,[29] Wen oversaw an emergency meeting of the State Council and warned that the country's economy, international image, and social stability might be damaged, and that "the overall situation remains grave."

The new sense of urgency and the notion that a new approach had to be taken was confirmed at a key Politburo meeting on April 17. This meeting marked a watershed in senior leadership response to SARS. Effectively, it acknowledged that China had been lying and called on officials to report periodically to the public (daily reporting had begun on April 1), not to delay reporting and not to cover up the situation. It also called for greater international and local cooperation and exchanging reports on experience in limiting the disease. It linked combating SARS to the policy line of the party congress, calling on each party committee and government to recognize the extreme importance of SARS work and to carry out prevention work through the realization of the "Three Represents."[30] The following day, it was reported that a new task force had been set up to oversee SARS work, now under the leadership of Beijing Party Secretary Liu Qi, a Politburo member.[31] Liu's deputies were Zhang Wenkang, the minister of public health; Meng Xuenong, Beijing's mayor; and Wang Qian, deputy director of the General Logistics Department of the People's Liberation Army (PLA).[32] The latter appointment clearly highlighted the need for better military-civilian co-operation.

The appointment of Zhang and Meng as deputies made it all the more surprising when they did not turn up for a press conference on April 20, which was run instead by Vice-Minister of Health Gao Qiang.[33] The conference was a public turning point in the Chinese leadership's attitude to dealing with SARS. Gao acknowledged that work had been lacking and that the fragmented jurisdiction over medical facilities in the capital had meant that accurate information had not been collected. In particular, he noted that it was difficult for municipal authorities to gather information on the epidemic from military-run hospitals, but observed that Hu Jintao and Wen Jiabao had remarked upon this. As a result, they had decided to put epidemic prevention work of all organizations whether party, government, or military under the leadership of the Beijing Municipal Government.[34] He also announced a number of other new measures. Unlike at Chinese New Year, it was now recognized that it was not a good idea to have tens of millions of people crossing the country for the seven-day May Day vacation, which was cut to one day. Supervision teams were to be sent out to investigate the situation in key provinces, and special concern was raised to prevent the disease from spreading into rural areas where the health system was liable to collapse. A special medical aid fund was to be set up to provide subsidies for those unable to cover the costs. The budget was to be shared between central and lower-level governments.

More dramatic than the press conference was the revelation that Minister of Public Health Zhang Wenkang, and Beijing Mayor Meng Xuenong had been relieved of their posts in a public display of ministerial responsibility for the mishandling of SARS. While not unprecedented, this was rightly interpreted as a dramatic move to acknowledge culpability and restore public trust, but not to undermine the party's credibility for having exacerbated the problems in the first place. To show the seriousness with which the leadership now viewed the "war," Vice-Premier Wu Yi was placed in charge of the ministry and was entrusted with overseeing policy. On April 23, a central command center was established headed by Wu, with a budget of 2 billion *yuan*.[35] Hainan Party Secretary Wang Qishan was appointed acting mayor. Ms. Wu is an experienced politician in China with good connections and a reputation for getting things done. She had worked with former Premier Zhu on WTO-entry terms and was not only considered well versed in Beijing politics but also had the trust of the foreign community.[36] Wang is one of the party princelings, being the son-in-law of Yao Yilin, but has an important reform track record of his own dating back to 1980, covering rural and financial sector work as well as provincial leadership. On April 30, he conducted a news conference that was screened live on television giving the impression of a new-style, straight-talking modern leader. He acknowledged that the health-care system was strained in coping with the disease, that citizens had been panicked by the outbreak of the disease, and that much needed to be done to ensure social stability. One of his first acts as acting mayor had been to order the building of a new hospital to deal with SARS, a hospital that was completed in record time.

However, the personnel changes did have a taint of factional intrigue attached to them. While it is clear that Minister Zhang had mismanaged developments, Mayor Meng seems to have been made a scapegoat. There were suggestions that Jiang Zemin would only accept the removal of Zhang, reportedly his personal physician, if Meng, who is thought to be close to Hu Jintao, was also removed. While the mayor stepping down to take ministerial responsibility may seem correct, in the Chinese political system, it is the party secretary who exerts supreme power and nothing can happen without his or her agreement. This would suggest that Liu Qi as party secretary would have been a more fitting sacrificial lamb. However, this was not possible for at least two reasons. First, Liu was a member of the Politburo and thus too important to be touched. Second, the party had tried consistently to absolve itself of blame, as in other incidents. Thus it was important to dismiss the mayor, a government official, while absolving the party of all culpability. Liu seems to have got away with a self-criticism, which in highly unusual fashion was reported in the official media on April 21. Liu acknowledged that he had provided inaccurate and late data and failed to contain the spread of SARS. "There have been obvious deficiencies in our work, I take responsibility of leadership and make a sincere self-criticism," he said.[37] At the same meeting, the head of the party's Organization Department criticized the municipality for its poor work, thus justifying the personnel changes.[38]

The dismissal of these two high-profile figures was accompanied by reports of 120 or more local officials being dismissed for failures in SARS work.[39] However, there was one very noticeable absentee from the list of dismissals, Guangdong Party Secretary Zhang Dejiang, who had overseen much of the original cover-up. Again the need to protect the name of the party probably aided Zhang, but the fact that he is a close supporter of Jiang Zemin's must have helped. His survival was ensured by the upbeat account that WHO officials gave on April 4 of the handling of the disease in Guangdong. They congratulated the Guangdong authorities for identifying the new disease and generally absolved them of their slow response.[40] This was subsequently used in late May as part of a counteroffensive to justify China's actions.

The energetic approach of Hu and Wen and the new appointments ushered in a brief period of unexpected cooperation and openness of reporting about SARS in the media. This not only helped warn the public of the dangers and allowed them to take sensible precautions but also indicated to other officials that they had to take SARS work seriously or face punishment. As in Guangdong, the disease peaked and new infections began to come down, helped by the stricter monitoring and reporting put into effect.

Restoring Politics as Usual

At the time, a number of observers were moved to optimism that this response might mark a fundamental change in China's political system and way of conducting business. However, the remarkable events were soon accompanied by conflicting signals and the reemergence of "politics as usual." While senior leaders such as Hu and Wen might have been convinced that "politics as usual" would not do, this view was not shared by all senior leaders. Nor was it signed onto by many local officials, who have become accustomed to particular ways of conducting business that do not include greater openness and transparency and use the latest campaign to pursue their own agendas.

Given that the crisis had domestic origins, it was natural that Hu and Wen would take the lead, but their energetic approach contrasted remarkably with that of former President and the then Chair of the Central Military Commission Jiang Zemin and his supporters. Jiang remained silent and his supporters invisible until April 26, when he met India's Defense Minister, George Fernandez, in Shanghai. His comments seemed strangely out of line with the national mood, noting that China had achieved notable achievements in containing the disease.[41] His remarks were much derided in the various mainland chatrooms and some suggested uncharitably that Jiang had fled to Shanghai to escape the threat of SARS. It did mark the start, however, of attempts by Jiang and his supporters to take a more visible role in the fight against SARS. His close protégé Zeng Qinghong went to the Central Party School on April 26 to tell them that it was "extremely important" that a regular teaching and study program be maintained,[42] this at a time when schools across Beijing were being shut down.

The residual influence of Jiang and his supporters was demonstrated at an April 28 Politburo meeting that again stressed the need to link the struggle against SARS with the need to promote Jiang's notion of the "Three Represents" and party building. The economic impact of SARS was also causing concern, given decreased consumption, which would be exacerbated by the cancellation of the May Day Holiday, and the concerns of foreign investors. Thus the fight against SARS was linked to the need to maintain economic development.[43] The theme was also taken up by Hu Jintao, who on a tour of Sichuan called on cadres to aim for a "double victory" in combating SARS and maintaining economic growth.[44] The military over which Jiang presided had been a major contributor to the confusion concerning the real state of the SARS epidemic, and its publications remained conspicuously silent. However, in a traditional move, on April 25, Jiang signed an order to send 1,200 army medical personnel to Beijing to help battle SARS. This was clearly intended to restore PLA prestige, which had taken a battering in recent weeks both domestically and internationally.

These developments went hand in hand with the traditional propaganda system getting to grips with the new demands. While the new campaign was geared to mobilizing people's support for the struggle against SARS, it was accompanied by more familiar restrictions on reporting. On April 25, the Propaganda Department met under its head Li Changchun to plot a new approach. He acknowledged the predicament that China was in because of SARS and stated that it was "more necessary for us than ever before to enhance our great national spirit."[45] The following day, the Propaganda Department highlighted the importance of Jiang's "Three Represents" in struggling against SARS and called on the nation's propaganda units to push the "great national spirit" in the struggle and victory over SARS.[46] This was more familiar ground, and the media began to be filled with patriotic gestures and accounts of individuals struggling against heroic odds and making personal sacrifices to defeat SARS. Traditional CCP language now took over. While the language of Leninism is that of struggle, the language of the CCP is that of war, and sure enough on May 1, Hu Jintao indeed declared that China was engaged in a "people's war" against SARS, for which the "masses should be mobilized."[47] This recourse to traditional propaganda techniques and the tools of mass mobilization disillusioned many who thought that SARS might herald real change, but they were effective in restoring party morale and dealing with the epidemic. In fact, Party Secretary Liu Qi saw the lifting of the travel advisory ban as a victory for national spirit.[48]

Constraints on the media were soon put back in place and the limited openness around SARS did not spread to other areas, despite optimism caused by the unexpected reporting of a major submarine accident that had resulted in the deaths of seventy sailors. By mid June, the Propaganda Department was clearly worried that the relaxation might go too far and moved to censure some publications while calling for all publications to stop reporting on sensitive topics.[49] This included writing stories critical of how Guangdong handled SARS and reporting about Dr. Jiang Yanyong who had brought the government cover-up to international and domestic attention. By the end of June, media outlets and academics had been warned not to analyze how the government had dealt with SARS. This was apparently prompted following the appearance of a sociology professor on China Education Television in early June, who had systematically analyzed government shortcomings.[50] This was in marked contrast with mid May, when a senior official from the Beijing Municipal Party Committee announced that "media have the right to expose any cover-up or false report on the epidemic situation" and referred positively to Dr. Jiang Yanyong.[51]

This followed the general pattern of reluctance to allow open discussion and has even led to those who have reported honestly coming in for criticism and official rebuke. For example, the Guangzhou-based *Southern Metropolitan News* was the first to report on SARS in February, but its editors and parent company were censured. The *Southern Weekend*, based in Guangzhou, had also earlier run into trouble. It was prevented from reporting about conditions in Shanghai on April 24 and was told that all SARS stories from outside the province could only be based on official sources such as Xinhua and the *People's Daily*.[52] The openness concerning reporting of SARS did not extend to the spread of other infectious diseases, such as Encephalitis B and HIV/AIDS. Further, the June 20 edition of *Caijing* magazine was withdrawn from the newsstands for its coverage of SARS and a political corruption scandal that was brewing in Shanghai.[53]

There were also attempts to exonerate key individuals and the party in general. At a press conference on May 30, Vice-Minister of Public Health Gao Qiang startled those present by defending the sacked Minister Zhang, claiming that he was still offering many good suggestions for work, denying that China had covered up the extent of the SARS outbreak and questioning why people were interested in Dr. Jiang, who had sounded the alarm. He had stated "I do not agree that Comrade Zhang Wenkang was relieved of his duties for concealing the situation of the epidemic. The Chinese government did not conceal the truth."[54] In Gao's view, Zhang had simply "lacked sufficient information at the time."[55]

This appears to have been part of a concerted attempt to deflect criticism and push the view that the government and its officials had not acted improperly. Gao blamed the institutional fragmentation of the system for preventing accurate reporting, while others blamed the difficulties in identifying a new disease. The head of the Beijing Propaganda Department, Cai Fuchao, acknowledged that statistics were inaccurate but insisted there was no cover-up. In contrast, he felt that "we have fully ensured the broad masses' right to knowledge of the epidemic and of work in other areas."[56] It was also reported that Jiang Zemin on a visit to Beijing had been seen drinking tea publicly with Zhang Wenkang. The *Economic Observer* was also apparently censured for criticizing Zhang's performance and Gao's attempts to belittle Dr. Jiang.[57] This appeared to herald a possible rehabilitation for Zhang, but at a conference on June 12, Gao was forced to acknowledge that the State Council had "made the decision, and the facts have proved that decision was entirely correct."[58] In Guangdong, officials even suggested that the disease had not originated in China but had been present in the United States in February 2002.[59]

Chinese authorities concerned about the use of new technologies to spread unauthorized views arrested 107 people in the second week of May for sending rumors by text messaging services to mobile phones.[60] The "war" on SARS has also been used to fight some old battles. Falun Gong was attacked for holding up SARS prevention work. It was claimed that Falun Gong followers had refused treatment and had tried to cause unrest at treatment facilities. The group was criticized for its "evil intentions of anti-mankind, anti-science, and anti-society" and wishing to see China fail in the fight against SARS.[61] Last but not least, it seems that SARS has even been used to detain migrants who have complained about resettlement programs associated with China's massive Three Gorges Project. One report cited instances where residents of Gaoyang who complained about resettlement issues were put into SARS quarantine.[62]

Lessons Learned or That Should Be Learned

However official publications might rewrite history, it is clear that fundamental shortcomings in China's system of management and governance exacerbated the problem and got the party into the mess in the first place. This has been recognized in a number of pieces in the official press and other media and is reflected in a number of measures introduced by the Chinese government. While none of the policy responses amounts to a significant change in practice, if implemented they should enhance China's capacity to respond to future emergencies and to provide a modicum of increased transparency.

A number of thoughtful pieces have pointed out the out-dated mode of crisis management and the challenges that new information systems present.[63] The *China Youth Daily* pointed out that misleading the public even if for good reasons can only end in creating more trouble than is necessary.[64] This was a theme explored in one of the more complete critiques written by Xue Baosheng, a researcher at the Central Party School's Policy Research Center. He lamented the fact that government was not used to dealing with the open flow of information and was overly concerned that it might cause social panic and disorder. However, as the author notes, this led to a swarm of rumors and the kind of social panic that leaders sought to avoid. He claimed that some officials were more concerned with economic losses than people's health and safety and more preoccupied with saving face. Again, the result was the reverse of intention, resulting in public resentment and causing economic loss and damage to their public image.[65]

With the benefit of hindsight, there are five key lessons that China's leaders should take from the SARS outbreak, as this will not be the last such crisis that they will have to deal with. These five areas range from dealing with global integration to putting national systems in place to deal with crises effectively, to enhancing incentives for timely reporting, to paying greater attention to social development, and to new ways of dealing with information flows.

Global Integration

China's leaders need to understand what it means to be a global player. China's entry into the WTO following its agreement to sign two UN covenants on human rights in 1997 and 1998 would appear to signal the Chinese leadership's intent to be a part of the global community. By signing these agreements, China has implicitly acknowledged that international monitoring is justifiable not only for domestic economic practice but also for political behavior. Membership in the world community entails a number of obligations and expectations on the part of others about what constitutes correct, ethical behavior. China, like others, would like to derive the economic benefits of globalization without having to deal with the social and political consequences. However, in practice, while China clearly wants to be a respected member of the international community, it is deeply conflicted about how active a role to play in international governance, and few have thought about how the process of globalization might impact domestic governance. The fact that globalization has impacted domestic governance, and will continue to do so, is poorly perceived, other than in terms of the need to censure incoming information and cultural flows.

SARS reinforced for China's leaders the notion that it is impossible both to maintain an open system for business investment and to close off flows of information and refuse transparency. China's leaders have often used not upsetting foreign investors as an excuse to suppress bad news. However, foreign investors may draw the conclusion that accurate information and greater transparency might be more important for making investment decisions. It was, after all, foreign concern and pressure from the WHO and international media that prompted China's senior leaders to take SARS seriously and begin to engage in more open collaboration. One of the most clearly recognized impacts of SARS is on China's international image. The *China Youth Daily* approvingly quoted the international affairs scholar Pang Zhongying as saying: "The greatest damage to China caused by the SARS crisis is the loss of China's reputation. For a great world-class economy that is growing vigorously, China's national image is especially worth maintaining and improving. Repairing the mutual trust between China and the international community is extremely urgent."[66]

As a result of international concern, when Premier Wen went to a special summit of the Association of Southeast Asian Nations and China on May 1, he was suitably contrite. He appealed for international understanding and stated that the Chinese government clearly had a responsibility to the world as a whole and proposed the introduction throughout the region of measures to create confidence. He noted that the "Chinese leaders and people have learned a lot" from SARS.[67] However, evading difficult questions and avoiding providing problematic information has a long pedigree in CCP history.

The residual suspicion of the international community combined with China's desire to be seen by all as a successful and civilized member of the world community explains the contradictions in China's international behavior. This can lead to decisions that are described as principled in China but that appear petty to others. China needs to improve its understanding of international norms and needs to become more comfortable with the framework for international governance that it seeks to join. SARS highlights how many issues beyond the directly political and economic, such as environmental protection, drug smuggling, trafficking in women, and HIV/AIDS, need China's active participation to resolve. In turn, other nations need to incorporate China as a more equal partner and to build China's reasonable concerns into the architecture of international governance. China for its part needs to reduce its suspicion of hostile foreign intent and adjust its outdated notion of sovereignty to accept that some issues need transnational solutions and that international monitoring does not have to erode CCP power.

Building Systems for Crisis Management

As we have seen, China needs to set up systems at all levels that can deal with crisis management. The initial response to crisis is denial and cover-up, and the vertical and segmented structure of China's bureaucracy hampers effective action once it is called for. Initially, leaders in Guangdong did not feel any urgency to provide information to Beijing, thus undermining the government's capacity to act effectively. Neither did the military hospitals think that it was their responsibility to inform the civilian authorities. The CDC head, Li Liming, is even reported to have said, "If we controlled the military hospitals at the beginning, we never would have had this epidemic in Beijing."[68] The problem was recognized at the April 20 press conference that talked of the multiple jurisdictions under which the medical institutions fell. As Vice-Minister Gao noted at the April 20 press conference, the "loose administration system has caused lack of communication among hospitals: a failure to obtain accurate information on the epidemic and a failure to take very effective quarantine measures to prevent the disease from spreading."

In the Chinese system, it is notoriously difficult to gather information across different sectors. With respect to SARS, military reporting was a particular problem. It was not until after the sackings of Zhang and Meng on April 20 that the situation improved, and it is not clear that reporting was timely and comprehensive even then.[69] It was not until May that senior PLA officials such as the CMC vice-chairs Guo Boxiong and Cao Gangchuan began to make SARS-related inspection tours.[70]

China needs to develop a system that encourages cross-sectoral collaboration to provide comprehensive, integrated solutions. This is not just a problem related to SARS; very few if any local administrations have in place an effective crisis response network, something that the Ministry of Civil Affairs was concerned about before the SARS outbreak.[71] All too often different ministries or localities work in their own interests to undermine national policy. In October, Wu Yi complained that some local governments had still not carried out central government directions for formulating emergency plans.[72]

A major problem is that the MOH is an institutionally weak player; for example, the Guangdong and Beijing party secretaries outrank the minister. This makes not only policy coordination but also policy implementation difficult. Provincial health departments and local disease control centers have to report first to the local party authorities. Thus, when the Guangdong Party Secretary told provincial health officials that the "peak of SARS has passed" and that the situation was starting to be controlled,[73] why should they dissent? China often sets up ad hoc bodies that make decisions that cannot then be enforced or are subverted by agencies at the same level or at lower levels. Even court rulings are not necessarily applied because local party secretaries will outrank local judges and the court may have no authority over actions taken in different ministries. Thus it will not help much to set up the new Emergency Response Bureau if it is not given real bureaucratic power to enforce decisions.

The most recent example of conflicting interests within the bureaucracy that threaten to undermine the prevention of future outbreaks is the question of the trade in wild animals.[74] On June 3, the Guangzhou city authorities announced that they wished to move toward centralizing the slaughter of poultry to improve hygiene in wet markets.[75] This followed earlier directives in the city and Shenzhen to stop the sale and consumption of wild animals. Fines range up to 10,000 *yuan*. It is thought that the most likely origin of the disease is that it crossed from animal species to humans in southern China, the civet cat being seen as a most likely suspect. However, this has not yet been proven conclusively, and agricultural authorities and the Forestry Bureau have objected to the ban, in particular. The Forestry Bureau is involved in direct regulation of the rearing and sale of wildlife and has seen the development of this trade as a way to raise farmers' incomes, a primary policy concern of the government. They are reported to be considering pushing to lift the June ban, arguing that there is no proven link that justifies its continuation.[76] Of course, should there be another outbreak of SARS, it will be the MOH that receives the blame and not the Forestry Bureau. Under these circumstances, it is difficult to apply a coherent policy.

A number of steps have been taken in this regard. The initial steps were to set up leading groups but these are just short-term stopgap measures. However, in mid May it was announced that China would set up an Emergency Response Bureau under the State Council to act as a powerful new agency to deal with future health crises and natural disasters.[77] This bureau is modeled on the U.S. Federal Emergency Management Administration that was established in 1979 and in March 2003 was absorbed into the Department of Homeland Security. Bureau membership will comprise heads of key ministries and commissions and will be tasked with drawing up plans for dealing with future emergencies.

Another key step was the promulgation on May 12 of temporary regulations on dealing with health emergencies. These had been overseen by Wen Jiabao and approved on May 9 and were drafted in a record sixteen days. The six chapters and fifty-four articles dealt with outbreaks of infectious diseases, large-scale food poisoning, and other serious public health threats. They laid out general rules and guidelines for prevention, reporting, and so on. The guidelines call, for example, for national authorities to be told within four hours of a major outbreak and provincial governments within eight hours. They also call for setting up CDCs all the way from the central government down to the county level, something that will add to the fiscal burden of local governments.[78]

Enhancing Government Performance

China needs to create an incentive system to encourage local governments to be more transparent and accept greater accountability. There is very little incentive for local leaders to provide accurate data and reporting; it is much better to report no problems or present statistics that exceed targets laid down by higher levels. The lack of accurate data makes policy coordination tough. Since they are unsure what higher authorities may think, the first reaction of local governments is to delay or suppress information. SARS is the latest in a long line of disasters that have been ignored or dealt with only haltingly. Recent examples are the poisoning of schoolchildren in northeastern China by bad milk and the disgraceful cover-up of deaths in Henan caused by AIDS-infected blood. Only when brought to the attention of a senior leader does action start, by which time the situation has been needlessly exacerbated, and the problem must in any case be solved without damaging CCP credibility. The need to "save face" and preserve the image of party infallibility all too often takes precedence over saving lives.

The response in the SARS case followed the normal pattern, and while the removal of the minister of public health and the mayor of Beijing was dramatic, it was not unprecedented during the reform period. For example, Ding Guan'gen was dismissed in 1988 as minister of railways because of an appalling safety record. Being Deng Xiaoping's bridge partner enabled Ding to bounce back later as the head of the Propaganda Department, and it seems that Zhang's close relationship to Jiang Zemin similarly led some to try to protect him from too much criticism. The dismissals did provide the signal for other dismissals at lower levels, but there are no norms in place to make officials accountable and to accept responsibility for mistakes. Political connections can overcome involvement in even the most egregious of scandals. Perhaps the best recent example of this is the fact that Jia Qinglin, who oversaw Xiamen at the time of one of the biggest corruption scandals in PRC history, was promoted to the Standing Committee of the Politburo in November 2002 and to head the Chinese People's Political Consultative Conference in March 2003. While there is no sign that Jia himself was involved in the corruption, despite his wife's close connection to groups involved in it, his promotion does not send a very reassuring signal about accepting responsibility for events that happen on one's watch.

Increasingly, however, it is being recognized that greater transparency is necessary in the actions of local governments and that innovation will be necessary to provide a better framework for governance. Party officials have also raised the idea that innovation is necessary. Thus Beijing Party Secretary Liu Qi said at a party meeting that "Beijing will expand the orderly participation of Beijing residents in politics and the people's right to know," but he added "we will transform the will of the party into the will and action of all Beijing residents." Little thought seems to have been given to what might happen if the residents are not unanimous in their views or do not find the party's will acceptable. It has also been suggested that the party would experiment with a tripartite division of powers in Shenzhen, and the Fujian party secretary, Song Defu, advocated the expansion of grassroots democracy, beginning with community self-rule.[79] These measures might help, but unless incentives are changed for local officials, there will be a clear limit to how much citizens can influence the decisions made on their behalf and demand the right to information that is crucial to their well being.

Improving Social Development

China needs to integrate social development and economic development better. The pressures of SARS have revealed the inadequacies of China's public health system. While markets have produced fabulous economic growth, they have changed ownership structures and incentives for healthcare, resulting in highly unequal access, increased costs, and an emphasis on expensive curative care over preventive services. Good health services, especially for the rural areas, are not a luxury or something that can be attended to once a high level of economic growth has been achieved.

The problems of the noneconomic aspects of reform had already become a focal point of leadership attention before SARS, and concern for those who have not fared so well under reforms has been a constant refrain of the Hu-Wen leadership. They have been at pains to portray themselves as more open, efficient, *and* concerned about the plight of the poor. In the eyes of many, Jiang Zemin represented the interests of China's new economic and coastal elites, and in the latter years of his rule, there was increasing concern about inequality and the potential threat this might pose to stability. During the leadership transition, Chinese reports played up the fact that both Hu Jintao and Wen Jiabao had spent significant phases of their careers in poorer western provinces. This is in marked contrast to their predecessors Jiang Zemin, Zhu Rongji, and Li Peng, who had worked in the developed metropolis of Shanghai or in the central ministries and bureaucracy in Beijing. The implied message was deliberate: the new leadership would show greater concern for those who have not benefited equitably from the reform program.

The outbreak of SARS could provide Hu and Wen with the opportunity to push social development further, especially given that it revealed the weaknesses of the Chinese health system in coping with the SARS crisis. It is significant that at a January 2003 Rural Work Conference, the party called for the countryside to be accorded the highest policy preference and acknowledged that rural problems were more intractable than those of the urban areas.[80] The CCP decided that most of any additional funding for education, healthcare, and culture would be allocated to the rural areas. Perhaps most important, the Conference stated that it was necessary "to make further adjustments to the structure of national income distribution and fiscal expenditure." If this goes beyond allocating more funds as the economy grows to actually redistributing resources to the countryside, it would be an extremely significant policy shift. However, given the current power structure and the benefits the coastal areas enjoy, any substantive redistribution of resources will be strongly resisted. The fragilities of the system revealed by SARS might, however, help with this policy agenda.

Certainly, during the SARS crisis, the new leadership showed concern for trying to provide financial support for those who might not be able to afford treatment. Premier Wen promised on May 6, 2003, that there would be free treatment for China's rural dwellers. He urged all governments to provide free medication, food, and accommodation to all SARS patients, whether confirmed or suspected. To meet this objective, the Ministry of Finance allocated 90 million *yuan* to cover expenses in nine poorer provinces in central and western China.[81] This followed a May 1 circular from the Ministries of Health, Finance, Labor and Social Security, and Civil Affairs calling for patients with fevers to be treated immediately, without going through the normal registration process, and stating that they should be treated regardless of ability to pay. However, there were persistent reports of patients being turned away or being charged despite central government attempts to prevent this. Because of the problems with financing in the health sector and hospitals now operating on a fee-for-service basis, many localities ignored the instructions and charged fees or requested sizable deposits. In addition, some claimed that guidelines were unclear as to who qualified, and some patients who were found later not to have had SARS were charged for their hospitalization.

Thus, although the center may make any number of pronouncements and send out directives, without clear incentives, local government officials will downplay social and welfare issues. The need to raise revenue forces local officials to concentrate on short-term economic gains over longer-term social issues. In addition, major pressure comes from the political contract system and the performance contracts that local governments and officials have to sign.[82] The precise nature of the contracts varies across time and from place to place, but they do set out performance expectations that provide the basis for official evaluation. Each county will set out performance contracts for the mayors and party secretaries of the townships under their jurisdiction to sign. Then contracts are signed between the towns and townships and the functional departments under their jurisdiction and then finally between the heads of these functional departments and their work personnel. This weakens the capacity for comprehensive development by township governments and disfavors social development.

The targets are divided into a mixture of priority, hard, and soft targets. The priority targets are set nationwide and usually are more political or policy-oriented in nature. They would include, for example, the maintenance of social order, most recently including the eradication of the influence of Falun Gong practitioners, and, of course, meeting the targets for family planning quotas. The hard targets concern primarily economic ones set by the county for the township and would include meeting tax revenues and certain levels of growth. The soft targets tend to relate to questions of social development such as health, education, and environmental protection. Clearly, meeting the hard and priority targets is the most important goal, because failure to meet them will mean that the rest of the work for the entire period will be discounted and there will be no promotions, titles, or economic rewards distributed. If social development goals were also written into these contracts and given more weight, this would be a major step forward in changing local government incentives.

Dealing with Information Systems

The Chinese leadership needs to create a new system of information management. This is an issue that has been much discussed in the mainland press. As we have seen, SARS was exposed by an incensed military doctor disillusioned with China's public health officials and domestic media, who turned to the international press, which in turn mobilized international opinion to put pressure on China's leaders to act. There is a fundamental tension between a system structured to control and manage information flows and a society that is information savvy and "wired." Treating citizens as children who need to be spoon-fed information and only permitted to hear good news is no longer viable when urban elites are part of a global information community tracking down and trading information online. You cannot have a domestic system saying that there is nothing wrong while cyberspace tells China's citizens that there most certainly is a problem. It is not even a question of who is correct; it is dysfunctional. It is also dangerous and threatens to undermine the social stability desired by the leadership to ensure economic development. If there is no trust in domestic reporting, people will turn to foreign sources or listen to rumors, leading to greater levels of discontent and distrust. Denial and cover-ups work against the leadership's long-term interests.

The role of the media and information flows are areas that Hu seems to have singled out for reform, and he has been trying to make the media more effective and possibly even more open. Since taking over as general secretary, he has been trying to promote the view that the media should be used to monitor some of the problems in society. Li Changchun who oversees that propaganda system and the minister of propaganda, Liu Yunshan, have echoed this.[83] In late March, the Politburo echoed Hu's instructions that Chinese journalism should be "closer to the practical [world], closer to the people, and closer to life." Certainly, many working in the mainland media have been bridling to play a more aggressive, investigative role, and it has been much more difficult in recent years to bury scandals entirely. Both Hu and Wen encouraged the media to take a more active role during the SARS outbreak. For example, in May, Wen called for the need for "timely, accurate and comprehensive" dissemination of information.

Many media outlets took the opportunity to blame the extent of the crisis on the way in which information was controlled early on, as did some academics. "The current diversification of information technology and broadcasting methods that is accompanying deepening globalization calls for suitable modes for guiding public opinion. In the past, when the public's channels of information were narrow, to some extent the government propaganda policies of 'internal vigilance and outward calm' could prevent information about crises leading to unnecessary panic," three Tsinghua professors noted. However, modern communication technologies had rendered such an approach outdated.[84] Similar messages were also picked up in more official media, with *Study Times*, the paper of the Central Party School, commenting that SARS had been a "salutary lesson" and that outdated information control had only deepened the crisis. To win the trust and respect of the people, it stated, it was necessary to uphold people's right to be informed properly.

However, as in other areas, it is more likely to be commercial pressures that bring about change. With WTO agreements coming into force and many mainland official press outlets between a rock and a hard place financially, foreign investment begins to look very attractive. The financial problems of party-run papers were enhanced by the decision that, in order to reduce the financial burden on them, rural entities should not be obliged to take out subscriptions. This was a major blow, because most party publications can only survive because so many party and government offices are forced to take out subscriptions. The media outlets have the political connections and the networks that might be attractive to foreign investors, but they cannot compete in the market with many of the more popular journals and magazines (many of which it must be said are set up by these official papers as money-making subsidiaries).

The topic of media reform found its way onto the agenda of the Politburo in August. Hu Jintao chaired a "study session" to consider what issues might be involved in liberalizing the media. Hu noted that with increased international contact, there was an inevitable conflict between "traditional thinking" and modernization. As a result, new ways had to be found to expand the "culture industry."[85] The main objective will be to make the domestic media more efficient, and presumably more readable, without weakening party control over ideology. China's new leaders need to draw the lesson that for continued rapid economic growth, they must encourage high and open information flows, reduce coercion, promote transparency, and enhance accountability.

The advent of SARS revealed some of the key contradictions in China's development strategy, primarily that between its rapid economic growth and its lagging social infrastructure. However, it also revealed how reform of its politico-administrative system has not kept pace with China's increasing integration into the international community. This is especially true of information management systems and the transparency of local government organizations. The fact that SARS became such a global crisis, and that it was controlled so quickly once the system kicked in,[86] are both results of the legacy of a top-down command political system.

Certainly, when SARS was at its height and public distrust was deepest, confidence in the system was shaken. As one official is reported to have said, SARS was a "huge shock for the entire party, you can sense this at internal meetings, where the atmosphere has changed and people are expressing criticisms more freely. The SARS epidemic is forcing us to rethink the whole theoretical framework for government that was developed under Jiang Zemin."[87] This tallies with anecdotal conversations with urban Chinese colleagues and friends who moved from disinterest to annoyance at foreign reporting to disgust with their government once the truth began to be told. However, as things were brought under control, these feelings of anger dissipated, with many feeling the government had eventually done a good job.

It is unrealistic to think that something like SARS will lead to significant short-term changes in the way the Chinese political system works, but it has revealed certain fault lines between the people's desire to know and their leadership's desire to retain a monopoly on information. The idea that key information affecting the lives of China's and the world's citizens should be withheld to protect economic growth and to avoid social instability has been shown to be erroneous.

If SARS does not recur, or if it recurs and the new systems that have been put into place work and it is dealt with more openly and effectively than in the winter of 2003–4, this will have enormous benefits for the Hu-Wen leadership and will allow them to pursue their own agenda of political tinkering. In that case, we may yet see greater attention paid to the social problems that now beset China and the difficulties that face rural China. In addition, not a free but a more challenging press may result, and local government officials may be held to greater accountability. The new leadership needs to complete the transition of governing structures from those that oversaw a communist state and planned economy to those that can run a modern market economy and accommodate a pluralized society.

SARS shows that in doing this they will not be able to rely on traditional CCP methods for controlling the country and will be under considerable pressure to find new ways to manage the Chinese polity. It is clear that the forces of globalization will require both a considerable shift in the way the CCP governs the system and political reform that seeks to make the system not only more transparent but also more accountable. They will have to deal with a much more fluid domestic and international political order, where many of the key decisions affecting China will be taken by international organizations that will not respect the CCP's outdated notion of sovereignty. Given its record to date, this will be a significant hurdle for the current leaders to overcome.

CHAPTER FIVE

SARS and China's Economy

THOMAS G. RAWSKI

Appraising the likely impact of SARS on China's economy involves a dangerous foray into economic forecasting. Forward projections are particularly risky for China because of massive institutional change and unusual structural elements (for example, the extraordinary rise of domestic inequality), and because recent growth outcomes remain shrouded in controversy. I begin with observations about the economic and institutional background, examine available information about the immediate impact of the 2002–2003 SARS outbreak, consider the implications for analyzing China's economy, and then briefly address longer-term perspectives.

China's Economy and Statistics System on the Eve of the SARS Outbreak

China's immense boom of the past quarter-century is a major episode in global history. Beginning in the late 1970s, China experienced two decades of extraordinary growth that raised every indicator of material welfare, lifted several hundred million from absolute poverty, and rocketed China from near autarchy into unprecedented global prominence. Despite claims that standard data overstate the dimensions of long-

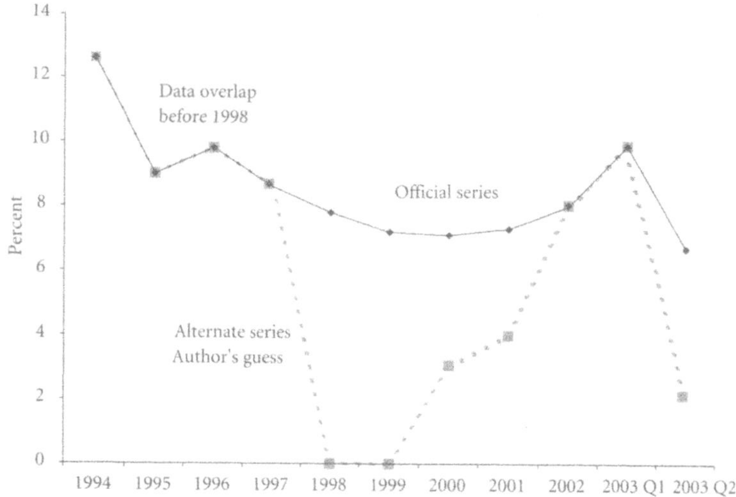

FIG. 5.1. Annual Growth of China's Real GDP, 1994–2003: Official figures and author's guesses (percent)

term growth, official statistics appear to provide a broadly accurate measure of national economic achievement during the first two decades of reform ending in 1997.

Broad agreement on economic performance terminates in 1997. Government statistics show growth continuing in the 7–8 percent range, but these figures appear to reflect official wishes rather than actual outcomes. In reality, China's growth slipped below the 7–8 percent range, especially during 1998 and 1999, when GDP growth may have fallen near or even below zero. This slowdown is partly attributable to the Asian financial crisis of 1997–98. The chief culprit, however, was domestic structural imbalance.

Figure 5.1 illustrates the gap between official performance data and this author's speculative estimates. Controversy continues over whether, and if so, by how much, official figures exaggerate performance during 1998–2001.[1] Critics, including the present author, argue that official growth claims clash with information about specific economic sectors and conflict with abundant evidence of a major slowdown in 1998 and 1999 followed by gradual recovery of momentum. Numerous Chinese commentators directly or indirectly questioned both the consistency and the veracity of official claims during the late 1990s.[2]

Events surrounding the SARS episode lend credence to the claim that official agencies have intentionally exaggerated China's economic performance. Alan Schnur and Erik Eckholm recount how Chinese officials sought to deny the severity of the SARS outbreak until a Beijing physician publicized accurate information. Stonewalling by top public health officials could hardly have occurred without the knowledge of China's national leaders. Against this background, the May 2002 complaint by National Bureau of Statistics Director Zhu Zhixin that "the statistics system cannot effectively resist intervention" invites the conclusion that orders from the highest levels may oblige official agencies to issue false claims about economic as well as health outcomes.[3]

When official data "lose touch with reality" (*shizhen*), to cite a common Chinese term, statistics agencies typically appear to be victims of political pressure rather than perpetrators of fraud. Indeed, China's National Bureau of Statistics (NBS) has worked diligently and effectively to improve China's economic statistics over the past quarter-century. While maintaining a steady flow of statistical information to policymakers, the NBS has familiarized its staff with internationally accepted methods of collecting and analyzing quantitative information, developed a system of regular household surveys, replaced Soviet-inspired systems with orthodox methods of national accounting, conducted a succession of national censuses, and developed a huge array of public information.

Despite these gains, and even without considering the "wind of falsification and embellishment" (*jiabao fukuafeng*) that rocked the statistics establishment beginning in 1998, it is widely agreed that the capacity of China's statistical authorities to produce accurate economic data has diminished over the past decade.[4] Expansion of China's market system has brought a reduction in public cooperation. Cost pressures and commercial secrecy have encouraged many entities to withhold data. At the same time, data collection networks have suffered from reductions in both personnel and budgets. The growing prominence of quantitative indicators in evaluating the performance of local government and party leaders compounds these difficulties.[5] When the incomes and career prospects of officials depend on data compiled under their own supervision, the temptation to manipulate crucial statistics is often irresistible—as is evident from information about American efforts to measure population, crime, aircraft reliability, and the number of student dropouts.[6]

Whatever the exact dimensions of China's recent slowdown, there is no dispute over the economic situation on the eve of the SARS outbreak. After slowly gaining strength during 2000 and 2001, China's economy enjoyed a banner year in 2002, sparked by a nascent automotive boom, a world record level of national steel output, massive foreign investment, and rising private business activity.[7] Rapid growth did not eradicate weaknesses that have burdened the economy in recent years: sluggish consumer demand, stagnation of farm incomes, slow employment growth. Despite these difficulties, China's economy steamed ahead during the first quarter of 2003 and appeared en route to another strong year until the unexpected arrival of SARS.

The Economic Impact of SARS: Short-term Effects

Historical experience indicates that direct economic consequences of one-time disease outbreaks are unlikely to extend beyond the short term.[8]

The broad outline of SARS's economic impact is clear. Calculations by Ren Ruoen, for example, indicate that seriously affected regions, including Guangdong, Beijing, and provinces adjacent to the capital, accounted for 22.7 percent of China's 2001 gross domestic product (GDP).

Peripheral regions accounting for 3.9 percent of GDP felt little effect from SARS. The remaining provinces, accounting for 73.4 percent of GDP, suffered only modest effects from the outbreak. Many accounts note that SARS mainly affected the tertiary or service sector, especially transport and communication, retailing, wholesale trade and catering. These hard-hit sectors accounted for approximately one-tenth of China's total output in 2001.[9]

These observations are not controversial. Despite occasional reports of factory closures, industry, the largest sector of China's economy, escaped major disruption. Official data for fifteen categories of industrial goods show output declining for eight items in May, five in June, and ten in July. Industrial value-added dropped slightly in May and again in July. Output of thermal electricity, a key measure of manufacturing operations, dropped by 4.4 percent in April, fell a further 2.0 percent in May, and then recovered slightly in June (when output remained 5.1 percent below the figure for April), followed by a big upward jump in July.[10]

Even though, as Ren Ruoen's analysis implies, the negative economic impact of SARS seems likely to be modest in scale and of brief duration, the politics of denial seems to have resumed control of China's national growth statistics in the second quarter of 2003. The predictable result was the announcement of statistics that strain credulity.

At the national level, official figures show that second-quarter GDP rose 6.7 percent above the comparable 2002 figure and 12.4 percent above reported output during the first quarter of 2003. The latter figure seems particularly improbable. The Chinese Entrepreneur Survey System's semi-annual poll of 2,000 companies found that "the volume of orders, production, exports and purchases all slipped during the second quarter" of 2003: "67 per cent of respondents said their orders dropped during the period, 67 per cent . . . said SARS increased their business costs and 65 per cent believe their profits have slumped."[11]

Disaggregation reveals further inconsistencies. The increase in completed fixed asset investment reported for the second quarter of 2003 is more than double the reported increase in nominal GDP.[12] The sum of quarterly changes in completed fixed asset investment, retail sales of consumer goods, and China's balance of merchandise trade (converted from dollars to renminbi at the official rate of Y8.28 = $1) is 46 percent larger than the reported change in total product.

SARS hammered China's entire retail sector. Damage was not confined to the regions with the largest concentration of disease victims: "Commercial sales dropped dramatically in the latter half of April following the outbreak of SARS in Beijing but a survey of 100 shopping malls across the country showed the sector to be recovering in May. . . . Sales. . . fell 35.66 per cent year-on-year in the first week of May, 24.39 per cent in the second week, and only 14 per cent in the third week."[13] Sales of electrical appliances during the spring "fell more than 45 per cent" in SARS-stricken regions of North China. "In other provinces, where the epidemic has had less impact, sales . . . fell an average 20 per cent."[14] A survey conducted in May found that "47 per cent of Chinese mainlanders claimed . . . to . . . have deferred major purchases in the past six months" on account of SARS.[15] With household incomes falling in rural areas, retail disruptions in the cities, airlines virtually grounded, and interprovincial travel subject to intermittent blockages, it is hardly surprising to read that "private consumption dropped 0.6 per cent in the first half of this year."[16]

Despite these (and many similar) statements, official data show that second-quarter retail sales were 5.3 percent above comparable figures for 2002—implying that sales of computers (+3 percent) and cell phones (volume and revenue down 3 and 10 percent respectively) lagged considerably behind overall retail sales![17] Retail sales typically drop between the first and second quarters. According to official data, the quarterly drop in 2003 (6.0 percent) was greater than in 2002 (1.2 percent) but smaller than in 2001 (6.4 percent). The implication that national retail sales during the SARS epidemic remained within the bounds of normal seasonal variation clashes head-on with overwhelming anecdotal evidence.

Among China's provinces, Beijing is uniquely dependent upon the service sector, which contributed 61.3 percent of the city's GDP in 2002, 10 percentage points higher than any other jurisdiction and 27 percentage points above the national average. The SARS outbreak prompted what Joan Kaufman describes as a "panic exodus" of students and migrant workers from the capital and essentially halted the normally huge influx of domestic and international travelers. As a result, Beijing's population dropped by perhaps 15–20 percent. Many public facilities and retail establishments closed their doors for several weeks. Despite these drains on economic activity, the municipality reported that total output during the first half of 2003 rose by 9.6 percent over the figure for 2002. Reported GDP for May was 4.8 percent above the figure for May 2002 and 14.4 percent above average monthly GDP for the first three months of 2003. Official reports place municipal GDP for the second quarter at 27.5 percent above results for the first quarter—more than double the comparable national figure, which shows a quarter-to-quarter increase of 12.4 percent.[18] These data indicate a local revival of the "wind of falsification and exaggeration."

As with 1998 and 1999, it is readily apparent that official data do not reflect actual economic outcomes. But what is the alternative? How badly did SARS actually hit China's economy?

At the moment, the market for petroleum products, which reflects activity throughout the economy, may offer the best insight into short-term fluctuations. Consider the following reports:

May 26: "China's second largest crude oil importer . . . is going to reduce the import of crude oil in [June and July 2003] by 8%. . . . One official from Sinopec revealed that the company has taken emergency measures to decrease the crude oil processing amount in the coastal refineries. . . . In May the processing amount in these refineries will fall by 10%. . . . At present, most regions in China have been hit by SARS, [and as a result] China's demand for oil product went down, and it is said that this effect will not disappear in a short time[;] as a result, the oil product market showed a descendent trend."[19]

June 20: "China's crude oil imports in May were the lowest so far in 2003 as state refiners slashed throughput to compensate for falling domestic oil demand due to SARS. . . . Falling domestic oil sales led China to churn out more barrels for export. . . . 'Everyone will agree that the reason is SARS, which hit Chinese domestic oil products sales and led refiners to cut output,' said a Beijing-based trader."[20] June 24: Two of China's largest refineries, Zhenhai [Zhejiang] and Qilu [Zibo, Shandong], plan to boost July production "due to expectations of a rise in domestic demand."[21]

June 27: "The third quarter will see a modest increase in China's oil products consumption as the threat of the SARS virus subsides, but demand still faces some pressure before returning to normal in the last quarter, a China-base[d] oil analyst said."[22]

July 2: "Singapore analysts predict that China's gasoline exports will rise in July 'as soft domestic demand prompted traders to export more cargoes.' These observers expect exports to fall in August due to 'reduced crude run rates [i.e., lower production] and a recovery in domestic demand in China.' "[23]

August 8: "China's second-largest refiner . . . is expected to reduce gasoline exports. . . . [according to a Beijing-based trader] 'We have problems now meeting the domestic demand, so exports for September are seen lower.' "[24]

With major refineries imposing "emergency measures" to scale back operations and diverting production to overseas markets because of the fall in China's demand for petroleum products, it is evident that, at the height of the SARS crisis, sales and consumption of petroleum products, and therefore the level of overall economic activity, experienced a steep decline. With pre-crisis growth plausibly reported in the vicinity of 9 percent during the first quarter, announcement of a 10 percent output decline by major refiners suggests that the crisis pushed the economy toward a temporary standstill during May and perhaps June, followed by a "modest" revival during the third quarter (amid continued reductions in refinery output) and expectations of normal market conditions (i.e., resumption of rapid growth) toward the end of the year.

Thus a plausible guess about China's economic growth during 2003 might include 9 percent expansion in the first quarter, a steep dive toward zero growth beginning in April and continuing into July, modest recovery during the third quarter and, further acceleration in the final three months.

The Economic Impact of SARS: Analytic Perspectives

Ren Ruoen has produced what may be the most systematic analysis of SARS's economic consequences.[25] Surveying various economic sectors, he observes that, as noted above, substantial negative consequences appear limited to specific segments of the tertiary or service sector, with other branches of the economy experiencing limited impact or, in the case of health services and pharmaceuticals, enjoying an unexpected boost to demand. In a worst-case scenario, Ren assumes zero output growth for the hardest-hit sectors—transport and communication along with wholesale and retail trade (including the catering industry). Since these sectors contribute approximately one-tenth of China's GDP, and with annual GDP growth anticipated to reach 9 percent in the absence of SARS, Ren concludes that a reduction of 0.9 percentage points (= 9 percent * 1/10) provides a generous upper limit to SARS-induced rollback of economic growth in 2003. Writing in June 2003, Ren anticipated actual GDP growth for 2003 of approximately 8.5 percent.[26]

This would represent a remarkable outcome. Economic history provides no instance in which a major economy has approached double-digit growth despite suffering a major crisis that caused activity to plunge in sectors employing massive segments of the labor force (restaurants, hotels, migrant workers) and in branches that maintain links across regions and industries (airlines, interprovincial transportation).

Regardless of the numerical outcome, the assumptions underlying Ren's analysis deserve attention. Ren projects national economic growth as a weighted average of sectoral growth rates, weighting each sector's predicted growth by its share in total output. If SARS reduces expansion in transport, catering, and trade to zero, as specified in the worst-case scenario, the overall effect, as noted above, is a reduction of 0.9 percentage points in national economic growth.

This approach, which ignores interactions that cut across sectors and regions, makes sense for evaluating the impact of small shocks—such as regional flooding or local damage from typhoons, drought, or insect pests. But the impact of SARS, although short-lived, was by no means marginal: official data show a steep drop-off in passenger transport, with May traffic reaching less than half of the March figures, and totals for July remaining more than 10 percent below the March results. The reported decline in freight traffic is much smaller, in part because official figures appear to underweight highway transport, which dropped by nearly one quarter between March and May and remained 5 percent below the March level as late as July.[27]

SARS-induced obstacles to the movement of people and goods were sufficiently large to attract the attention of editorial cartoonists. The *China Business Weekly* of June 24–30, 2003, depicted a combine harvester chained to a boulder labeled "Inter-provincial business forbidden to stem the spread of SARS." Can we assume that agriculture suffered no ill effects and that manufacturing was able to bound forward at double-digit rates despite steep declines in transportation and in wholesale and retail sales?

In the same vein, Ren's analysis discounts any consequences of widespread income losses for production, investment, or sales. It does not explore the implication of reports showing that "evaporated jobs for rural migrant workers in cities and limited access to urban markets for agriculture produce . . . when SARS peaked all significantly added to the pressures on farmers' incomes," which appear to have declined in recent years and reportedly dropped by RMB 35 per head during the second quarter,[28] or that less than one-fourth of the migrant workers who fled the cities to escape SARS had "returned to work in cities" by June 15.[29]

In essence, Ren's study visualizes the economy as an array of more or less self-contained units. Unexpected disruption affects only the sectors or regions directly involved, leaving the remainder to pursue an unobstructed path to fulfilling pre-shock expectations. Although I find it difficult to imagine that this perspective, which echoes the circumstances of a centrally planned system, fits China's increasingly marketized economy, Ren's approach mirrors a substantial body of international research that depicts China's economy as a collection of weakly connected boxes.

This emphasis on absence of economic integration dates from Audrey Donnithorne's 1972 article on "China's Cellular Economy," which argued that the economy "seems composed of a myriad of small discrete units. . . . [which] often provide a high degree of administrative protection . . . to home producers."[30] This tradition commands considerable support today, despite staggering multiplication of domestic and international commerce in the intervening decades.

A 1994 World Bank report shows the expansion of domestic trade lagging behind the growth of total output.[31] Christine Wong shows how official protection by local governments may lead to the proliferation of excess capacity, with sheltered factories operating below capacity.[32] Andrew Watson and others provide detailed accounts of provincial and local barriers to domestic commerce.[33] Alwyn Young finds that interprovincial differences in the composition of industrial output, notably small during the pre-reform plan era, have shrunk further during the reform era, presumably because China's provinces implement mercantilist policies intended to promote local self-reliance.[34] Sandra Poncet, working with provincial input-output tables, calculates that the share of local goods in provincial absorption, already high in 1992, rose further between 1992 and 1997, mainly at the expense of "imports" from other provinces.[35] Genevieve Boyreau-Debray and Shang-jin Wei conclude that the magnitude of interprovincial capital movement resembles flows across the boundaries of autonomous nations rather than domestic transfers of funds in integrated economies like Japan or the United States.[36]

Proponents understand that the cellular economy perspective remains controversial. Poncet remarks that "the claim of increasing fragmentation in China is received with skepticism by China specialists. Reports of rising regional trade barriers run strongly counter to the perceptions of informed observers. . . . Notably they fly in the face of the visibly successful efforts by both foreign multinationals and emerging Chinese enterprises to build national distribution networks and establish nationally recognized brands."[37] Authors advancing the cellular perspective understand that "overturning conventional wisdom [of China specialists] requires very solid empirical work" and take pains to offer detailed accounts of their analysis.[38]

Here I join the skeptics. I anticipate that future research will undercut the picture of China's economy as a loosely connected set of local systems. Dynamic new industries producing motorcycles, cars, computers, home appliances and an immense array of export goods display a high degree of regional concentration. Barriers to commodity trade appear episodic rather than systematic. Municipal officials can no longer exclude "imports" from other provinces. Manufacturers ridicule the suggestion that local politicians systematically prohibit inflows of low-priced, high-quality components and finished products. China's burgeoning network of expressways represents the latest element in a transport revolution that has multiplied the circulation of commodities, people, and information across China's vast landscape.

Transportation statistics provide an obvious starting point for revisionist research. If official figures understate the actual volume of traffic, domestic flows of commodities, people, information, and funds—the foot soldiers of economic integration—could be far larger than standard data have led cellular economy proponents to believe.

Underestimating traffic volume appears to be endemic. Robert W. Mead and I have speculated that standard data "grossly underestimate the level and growth of transport activity." For the 1990s, Ralph Huenemann found that standard data "fail to capture a significant portion of the traffic, and the problem seems to get worse as the decade progresses."[39] Difficulties cluster in two sectors: highways and water carriage.

As far back as the mid 1980s, Zhang Fengbo noted that with growing numbers of vehicles operating outside the network of official transport companies, "there is a vast underestimate of the actual haulage by motor vehicles, because the figures are based solely on freight haulage by the companies within the official transport system."[40] Subsequent revisions appear to have corrected this particular oversight, but a recent 30-fold increase in official estimates of the number of vehicles used for commercial transportation suggests the likelihood of continuing large-scale underestimation of highway carriage.[41] Private ownership or management of trucks and buses creates strong incentives for systematic underreporting of revenues (which attract taxation) and hence volumes: since individual entrepreneurs "keep no proper accounts, revenue and cost, profit and loss reside only in the mind of the operator, which creates grave difficulties for supervisors and tax collection and translates into big fiscal losses."[42]

Standard sources are filled with improbable data that confirm the diagnosis of underreporting. Construction of a growing network of expressways has not raised the share of highway carriage in official freight statistics—the reported share actually declined from 14.4 percent in 1998 to 13.3 percent in 2001 and 2002—a level scarcely above the 12.8 percent reported for 1990.[43] Successive issues of China's national statistics yearbook indicate that highway freight haulage in Sichuan province peaked in 1995, the first full operating year for the expressway connecting the two major cities of Chengdu and Chongqing. Comparing the data for 1995 and 2001, we discover that the combined truck fleet for Sichuan and Chongqing (which was promoted to provincial status in 1997) increased by 65.4 percent, while highway freight carriage (measured in ton-kilometers) declined by 21.5 percent, which implies that average haulage per vehicle dropped by 52.5 percent.

Figures for water transport are equally suspect. Official data show the scale of water carriage growing slowly, with periodic annual declines—the tonnage of waterborne freight, for example, recorded a peak in 1996, which was not surpassed until 2001. The figures also show a large decline in both the overall number and, more improbably, in the number of privately owned motor vessels and barges.[44]

In 1996, when statistics showed that "water freight slipped 1.5 percent," the Ministry of Communication "suspended approval of new shipping companies to slow uncontrolled growth in waterway transportation."[45] This pattern continues, with slow growth of reported freight volume and fleet size coinciding with complaints of "blind entry into the market for water transport."[46] Reports of unlicensed vessels offer further evidence of underreporting: investigations around Changzhou, in Jiangsu province, found that two-thirds of vessels were not properly licensed; the proportion of gypsy craft was even larger on the Yangzi River.[47] Existence of numerous shipyards—ninety-six in Sichuan alone—supports the view that, contrary to standard data, shipping fleets continue to expand.[48]

SARS dealt a brief but sharp setback to China's economy. The immediate decline in output occurred primarily in the tertiary or service sector and mainly during the second and third quarters of 2003, followed by a short-lived drag from slow export growth (orders for future output declined during the epidemic), higher inventories, and "increased employment pressure" because "many small and medium-sized enterprises suspended their operations or simply closed down, which... aggravated the already acute employment contradiction."[49] Fortunately, the hangover from SARS failed to affect foreign investment.

The SARS episode seems to have sparked at least a temporary return to the pattern of systematic overstatement of economic performance that emerged during 1998–2001.

Efforts to anticipate the economic impact of SARS focus attention on a surprising convergence of scholarly opinion linking immense economic growth with minimal progress toward domestic economic integration. Systematic studies by authors like Kumar, Wong, Young, Poncet, Wei, and Boyreau-Debray appear to demonstrate the limited extent of domestic economic integration. Against this substantive body of work, evidence supporting the contrary, "integrationist" perspective remains scrappy and unsystematic.[50] Nonetheless, I venture to predict that further study of China's market structures, division of labor, and interregional flows of goods, people, and funds will reveal a very substantial degree of integration. Despite remaining obstacles, as when "strong concept of planned economy. . . . too much government interference. . . . inconvenient traffic network and serious regional barriers" create "duplicated construction" and allow only a "sluggish economic integration process" in the region adjacent to the Bohai Sea,[51] I anticipate that such research will provide convincing evidence that, whatever its merits in illuminating circumstances during the 1970s, the cellular economy perspective cannot provide a suitable framework for analyzing China's present-day economic system.

The SARS episode permits broader observations about China's economy and society: dynamic economies can survive substantial shocks without losing their momentum. China's economy plowed through the 1989 Tiananmen massacre and the 1997 Asian financial crisis. Recovery from SARS will again confirm the deep roots of Chinese economic growth.

SARS provided an unexpected test of electronic networks as substitutes for the personal interactions that normally precede business deals. The results were mixed: in textiles, export orders dried up during the crisis, but elsewhere electronic technology provided an unexpectedly good substitute for face-to-face encounters.

SARS shows that Chinese governments routinely ignore legal requirements. China's 1989 Law on Prevention and Control of Contagious Disease prohibits concealment or distortion of information (Art. 22) and states that the "Ministry of Health should make timely and accurate public reports" about contagious disease conditions (Art. 23).[52] Neglect of legal obligations is not unusual: the Aluminum Corporation of China anticipates that "local governments are likely to seek more investors to accelerate the development of their alumina resources" even though the corporation "signed agreements with [those same] local governments giving it exclusive rights to develop ore resources."[53]

SARS also highlights beneficial aspects of authoritarian government. If we consider China's limited medical capabilities, it would appear that the People's Republic (and also Singapore) controlled the epidemic more effectively than Hong Kong, Taiwan, or Canada, apparently because China and Singapore did not hesitate to implement stringent quarantine regimens—measures that governments operating under individualist traditions cannot readily deploy.

Finally, SARS demonstrates China's progress toward achieving a more open society. The Nobel laureate A. K. Sen has often emphasized that India's free press would prevent New Delhi from suppressing news of a national tragedy in the way that Beijing concealed the reality of China's 1959–61 famine.[54] Although Sen is right about the Great Leap, times have changed. Chinese publications took only a few months to denounce the 1998 deluge of false economic data. More recently, public pressure has forced China's health authorities to recognize China's growing AIDS problem. And in 2003, official efforts to deny the realities of SARS collapsed abruptly. All this shows how two decades of reform have dramatically curtailed the capacity of China's government to control the dissemination of important but unwelcome information.

CHAPTER SIX

SARS in Beijing

The Unraveling of a Cover-Up

ERIK ECKHOLM

The Cake Was a Tip-off

On April 3, 2003, months after a fearful new pneumonia first appeared in southern China, debilitating Guangdong and Hong Kong, and with rumors swirling that it had invaded Beijing, China's central government held its first press conference on SARS.

Journalists arrived to find an elaborate spread of cakes, pastries, tea, and coffee—an unusually generous offering for a press conference—that immediately raised suspicions. The event was being televised live, a sign that the government had an urgent message for the public.

The Information Office of the State Council, or cabinet, invited foreign and domestic journalists to hear the minister of health, Zhang Wenkang, and the mayor of Beijing, Meng Xuenong. The officials were confident, even smug, in demeanor. "Look at this room. All of you are still in Beijing, not afraid to enter a crowded room, and few of you are wearing masks," Mayor Meng said. "So you all know there is no SARS problem in Beijing."

"SARS in our country is under control," said Zhang. "I can responsibly tell people now it is safe to live, work, and travel in China."

According to Zhang, SARS cases had peaked in Guangdong. This claim was endorsed by a World Health Organization team, which was finally allowed to visit Guangdong this same week. However, a second assertion was met with popular disbelief, triggered outrage abroad, and would prove to be the officials' personal undoing. Officials insisted that only 12 cases had appeared in Beijing; and that all of these cases were "imported." In other words, patients had contracted the virus elsewhere and there was no local transmission.

According to government statistics reported that day, China's SARS cases as of March 31 totaled 1,190. Of these, all but 47 cases were in Guangdong; and there were only 46 fatalities.

During that same week in early April, as the May Day holiday approached, national officials urged continued domestic tourism and travel. The May Day holiday is traditionally a time of heavy domestic travel. "A well-organized holiday, with millions of people traveling around this vast country, will show the world that tourism in China is secure and healthy," said Sun Gang, deputy director of the National Tourist Administration. This pronouncement, that holiday travel should not be affected, would soon be seen as irresponsible and reversed.

The official bravado convinced no one. Many Beijing residents had heard stories of friends or relatives who were seriously ill and quarantined in hospitals. True and untrue reports of SARS cases flew via text messaging on mobile phones. Largely true stories were passed along about doctors and nurses who had disappeared from view, and hospital wards that were suddenly off limits.

Some Chinese doctors had reported privately to Chinese and Western journalists a few weeks earlier that there were hidden clusters of SARS patients in Beijing, and that orders had been issued to keep such clusters secret. News reports printed abroad quickly found their way back to China via the Internet.

One person who watched the April 3 press conference on television was Dr. Jiang Yanyong, a senior doctor (aged 71) in the prestigious military hospital system. Dr. Jiang had firsthand knowledge of the emerging epidemic in Beijing. He was so outraged by the official claims that he took the risk of speaking out to Hong Kong and Western media outlets. In an initial letter, Dr. Jiang said he personally knew of more than 60 SARS patients and numerous deaths in Beijing military hospitals. In subsequent telephone interviews, Dr. Jiang said he knew of over 100 cases.

Although the Chinese press was not allowed to report Dr. Jiang's assertions, Beijing residents soon learned of them. The public awareness of Dr. Jiang's reports emboldened journalists and international officials to question the official line. At this time the World Health Organization, with some fairly strident public comments in Geneva and quiet negotiating in Beijing, pressed its request for an official visit to Beijing medical and public health facilities. One implicit club it wielded was the possibility that Beijing and other regions of China could be added to the WHO travel advisory, joining Guangdong and Hong Kong, a step the Beijing government was anxious to avoid. (Beijing would soon be added in any case.)

In a second press conference on April 10, officials raised the city's case total to 27 and, in response to questions, explicitly stated that this number included patients in both military and civilian hospitals. The lack of credibility was evident on the streets, where more people donned protective masks and shopping center crowds rapidly dwindled. Significant numbers of expatriates, including families of Western diplomats, began to leave the country.

As foreign condemnation and public disbelief—bordering on outrage—grew, signs of high-level party and government policy changes appeared in mid April. President Hu Jintao made a much-publicized trip to Guangdong, where he visited a hospital treating SARS patients, a clear step toward more openness. Deputy Prime Minister Wu Yi began making private inquiries of Beijing medical officials and met with WHO officers.

Actually revealing the truth about the extent of SARS in Beijing and elsewhere in China would take a bit more time and some political finessing. With foreign and domestic pressures rising, the government approved an initial WHO evaluation of Beijing. Top officials must have known that the WHO team would find serious underreporting of SARS cases and disarray in infection-control programs. However, for Communist Party leaders confronting an embarrassing and politically sensitive reversal, this approach may have been seen as the most palatable way to proceed—to ease their way from a posture of denial to one of chagrined discovery, and then forceful action.

On April 16, after their first few days of site visits in Beijing, a WHO team of epidemiologists and virologists met with foreign journalists. In an apparent attempt to avoid humiliating or angering Chinese leaders, who were contemplating how to reverse their policies, the WHO team spoke only in the most general terms about serious gaps in Beijing's tracking and SARS control measures. Members of the team said they had insisted on visiting key military hospitals and found SARS cases, but that they had been allowed in on the condition that they not publicly reveal what they saw.

Prodded by a frustrated crowd of journalists, Dr. Henk Bekedam, the WHO Beijing director, said the team had found Dr. Jiang's assertions about large caseloads "very credible." Dr. Alan Schnur, chief epidemiologist in the Beijing office and a team leader, said of Beijing's total cases, "My guess is that we are in the 100 to 200 range now." This, he later admitted, was an underestimate, but in the context of this press conference it was a bombshell: the firmest confirmation yet that the Chinese government had dangerously misled its public and the world.

On April 19, journalists received an urgent invitation to another press conference the following morning at the State Council Information Office—again to meet with the health minister and mayor, or so the invitation said. But reporters arrived on April 20 to find a new, hitherto unknown, cast of speakers. At that moment it was apparent that the government had turned an important corner. No one bothered to explain the mysterious absence of the advertised speakers and no one had to. (At about the same time, the Xinhua news agency announced that Zhang and Meng had been relieved of their duties.) Before live television cameras, the newly appointed deputy health minister began the distasteful and touchy process of coming clean.

Gao Qiang, a seasoned bureaucrat with more of a financial than a health background, announced that Beijing had 339 confirmed and 402 suspected SARS cases. Furthermore, not only were the numbers climbing daily, but more than 200 patients receiving treatment in the city's military hospitals had been omitted from previous case reports.

Neither Gao nor other senior officials admitted that the government had engaged in intentional concealment. Instead, Gao made the less damning claim of confusion: "The Ministry of Health was not adequately prepared to deal with a sudden new health hazard." He did, however, suggest that top officials had been kept in the dark: "Accurate figures have not been reported to high authorities in a timely manner."

Gao said that a key problem was the many different political jurisdictions governing hospitals in the capital city. He promised that henceforth, all patients, from both civilian and military facilities, would be included in the daily case totals. He said that the upcoming May Day holiday would be shortened and travel severely curtailed.

Once the top leaders recognized the political and medical dangers and saw transparency as their only way out, they swiftly enacted sweeping measures. Although the two dismissed officials were not publicly excoriated, their fates sent a message down the ranks. The long-muzzled media were ordered to give extensive coverage to SARS risks, and to emphasize the heroism of doctors and nurses, invariably referred to as "white angels." Twice a week for several weeks, Beijing officials held televised press conferences where they endured probing, often embarrassing questions from foreign journalists, which would later be recounted with glee by some Beijing residents.

The new countermeasures sometimes seemed excessive or irrational, but overall, they had the desired effect. Thousands who had possible contact with SARS carriers, including college students and apartment dwellers, were quarantined in their homes or, in some cases, in special centers. The elderly legions of the Neighborhood Committees were out in the streets with their red armbands, watching to keep strangers or sick-looking people from entering residential compounds. The city's schools were closed.

Surrounding villages erected barricades to prevent nonresidents from entering and ensure a temperature check for residents as they came and went. At the gates of many villages and compounds, people in protective gear sprayed disinfectant on the tires of all vehicles passing through—a measure sometimes used to control animal diseases—but with no logical impact on SARS transmission. If nothing else, these various measures, reminiscent of Maoist mobilization, did serve to raise awareness and make more people feel involved in the battle.

For a few weeks, new SARS cases in the city climbed by a hundred daily. Stores were virtually deserted and the subways sparsely ridden. Only a few forlorn-looking migrant workers, carrying their belongings in sacks, rode the subways to train or bus stations as they fled back to their villages. Some left due to fear of disease; others because their jobs in tourism, recreation, and most construction had come to a temporary halt.

At bus and train stations, airports, and even many building entrances, medical stations were set up to take the temperatures of all who passed, or at least purported to do so, often with instruments of dubious value. It is unclear how many actual SARS carriers were detected with these procedures, but anyone with a visible cold or a high fever definitely got the message: stay at home or risk medical detention.

It is not hard to understand the combination of international and domestic political, economic, and medical factors that compelled China's senior leaders to end the dissembling and start fighting SARS widely and openly. As the virus quickly spread throughout Beijing, Shanxi province, and Inner Mongolia, the risk seemed real of a runaway epidemic both in major cities and smaller towns with generally poor medical capacities. The exodus of expatriate families and cancellations of business visits and conferences signaled the potentially devastating effect on foreign investment and economic modernization.

The blow to China's international credibility and prestige was already profound and had somehow to be repaired. Hong Kong residents in particular felt they were victims of China's initial secrecy, and questions were raised regarding the wisdom of holding the 2008 Olympics in Beijing. At home, popular disillusionment, suspicion, fear, and anger were rising—factors that today's leaders must think about.

The role of the WHO in shepherding the policy turnabout should make an interesting case study of the changing nature of international power. The agency's public complaints and private interventions, the threat of extended travel sanctions and finally the offer of technical aid all played roles. By April, the WHO possessed tremendous leverage: a breakdown in cooperation or even more forceful international condemnation of the Chinese government would have had devastating consequences for the country. At the same time, once the leaders did change course, they made use of the WHO's involvement to reassure the public.

Still unclear is the role of senior party and government officials in the repeated efforts to cover up the extent of SARS. SARS entered Beijing in early March. Did Hu Jintao and Wen Jiabao know this and approve the strategy of concealment, perhaps to avoid disturbing the National People's Congress that month at which the two were named to the posts of president and prime minister? Or did lesser officials take this path without asking? Did the top leaders realize how duplicitous the health minister was on April 3?

Given the earlier events in Guangdong, where initial efforts to downplay SARS backfired, senior leaders were at a minimum seriously negligent, in my view, even if they were simply poorly informed and failed to focus on the SARS threat. True, confusion and incompetence may have left even the health minister unsure about the true scale of the spiraling epidemic. But the repeated orders of secrecy came from somewhere on high. And it is impossible to maintain, to take one example, that the mayor of Beijing (who was deputy party secretary of the city) would have acted so strenuously to conceal SARS without consulting his immediate boss, Liu Qi, who remained party secretary of Beijing, as well as a member of the Politburo, and escaped with a quick public apology.

In many countries, a similar deadly fiasco might overturn the government. In China, government credibility was low to begin with, and my impression, based on widespread interviews in May and June of 2003, is that President Hu and Prime Minister Wen were, on balance, personally strengthened by the events, even if broader trust in the system sank to a new low. Their counterattack on SARS, if belated, came across as strong and in keeping with the image the new leaders had cultivated of being more in touch with "the people" than their predecessors. The sacrifice of two officials, even if they were widely seen as scapegoats, helped to satisfy many people's desire for accountability. Most important, the leaders benefited from their apparent success in quelling the disease.

China's rulers learned a hard lesson about the dangers of secrecy and a controlled press, at least when infectious diseases are involved. Yet, despite hopes expressed by some Chinese and foreign observers in late April, there has been no evidence of a move toward more freedom in the media. The new instructions were to cover SARS extensively, but these were still instructions, with permissible themes dictated by the central Propaganda Department. Riots in several locations around the country linked to plans to establish SARS treatment or quarantine facilities in unwilling communities were never reported by the Chinese media.

Although for a brief time a few newspapers printed laudatory articles about Dr. Jiang, certainly one of the true heroes of the story, the major party newspapers did not do so, and he has never received official praise for his candor. He was not jailed for breaking ranks, but he did receive warnings to stop talking to the press.

Not long after the awkward revelations of April 20, the Propaganda Department found a new voice and sought to turn this near-debacle into a triumph for the leaders, the party, and the nation. "In the Midst of Disaster, the Unity of the Masses is an Impregnable Fortress," read a page one headline of the *People's Daily* on April 24.

On May 15, in a typical continuation of the campaign, the *People's Daily* carried a front-page commentary titled: "Build Our New Great Wall—On the Great Spirit of the Fight Against SARS." In the struggle against this new disease, the party's flagship newspaper said, "the party central leadership with Hu Jintao as general secretary" had proved its "concern for the people, determination and maturity, ability to master complex situations, and ability and boldness to deal with severe challenges."

"The people have become more trusting and supportive of the party and the government," it concluded. So much for a new spirit of open debate.

PART III

Social, Moral, and Psychological Consequences

CHAPTER SEVEN

Psychological Responses to SARS in Hong Kong—Report from the Front Line

DOMINIC T. S. LEE
AND YUN KWOK WING

> This is not real. This is not real. This is not real. Then I'd shake myself. Damn right it's real, and I had better figure out what I'm going to do about it.
>
> —Rudolph Giuliani

In many ways, the emotional responses to SARS during the 2003 outbreak were not different from the emotional responses to September 11, 2001, so vividly captured by Rudolph Giuliani in his memoir *Leadership*. Much as New Yorkers had not envisaged the terrorist attack, most Hong Kongers had not imagined being involved in a life-threatening epidemic. When SARS arrived on Hong Kong's doorstep, we had no idea that we were facing a major disaster that would for months permeate and overwhelm the daily, lived experiences of every segment of the population. Many people were initially plagued by a sense of doubt and "unrealness"—that it could not be true that Hong Kong had been struck by a new virus, previously unknown to mankind. But before long, as the outbreak swiftly unfolded, morbidity and mortality escalated, and the society came to a standstill, we could no longer deny that we were in the midst of a historical epidemic, and that we had to do something about it. The authors—both academic psychiatrists who became involved in the SARS crisis in one way or another—naturally chose to study the psychological responses of Hong Kong society to the disaster.

The emotional experiences of living through the SARS outbreak were profoundly rich and intense. Capturing the psychological impact of the epidemic is hence extremely challenging. Many of the outbreak experiences are truly beyond words, and summarizing the psychological responses in numbers is no simple task. The authors of this chapter hope to retrace the fear and panic, the helplessness and bewilderment, the frustration and anger associated with the SARS outbreak using an ethno-epidemiological approach—putting quantitative and qualitative findings side by side so that the ethnographic observations and insights can inform the figures and statistics, and vice versa.

During the SARS epidemic, one author of this chapter (YKW) and his colleagues carried out a number of quantitative studies. Using psychological paradigms and research instruments, they studied how the general public and SARS patients responded to the catastrophic outbreak. They asked what proportion of the population or SARS patients developed psychiatric disorders, and what would increase their vulnerability to decompensation.

The other author of this chapter (DL), who had prior training in medical anthropology, decided to initiate an ethnographic study of the outbreak. The qualitative enquiry consisted of two parts. The first was a general ethnography based on material and information collected from newspapers, magazines, radios, books, photos, television, films, web sites and Internet chat room discussions, as well as monographs dedicated to SARS in Hong Kong, China, and other parts of the world. The second part of the ethnography was a participant observation conducted by DL who lived through the entire SARS epidemic in Hong Kong. Being an academic clinician who had outpatient sessions at the Prince of Wales Hospital, one of the epicenters of the outbreak in Hong Kong, DL was well positioned to conduct the participant observation.

Through psychiatric epidemiology, general ethnography, and participant observation, the authors strive to represent the lived experience of the SARS outbreak. What was it like to be living through a modern epidemic? What was the population psychology in response to a public trauma? How and why do people succumb to the dread of SARS? The authors also seek to use the epidemic as a lens through which to examine the postcolonial sociopolitical landscape and how the SARS outbreak drove half a million Hong Kongers to demonstrate on July 1, 2003.

The Spread of SARS and the Spread of Fear

At dusk, on March 10, 2003, DL met one of his neighbors, a microbiologist, in the university residence car park. They chatted as usual, and the microbiologist casually mentioned that there was a small outbreak in one of the medical wards. Nearly a dozen doctors and nurses had taken ill, and the internists and microbiologists were busily looking for the culprit pathogen. We parted, hardly realizing that that was the last relaxed moment we would share for months to come. Neither of us had ever imagined that Hong Kong might become the epicenter of a deadly global outbreak.

The SARS outbreak had begun months earlier in Foshan City, Guangdong. A chef working regularly with game meat was admitted for pneumonia with atypical features. He was later identified as the first SARS case. In the subsequent months, SARS spread to other cities and provinces in China, but Guangdong province remained the most severely affected. By February 11, according to the formal report dispatched by the Chinese Ministry of Health to the World Health Organization (WHO), 305 persons (including 195 health-care workers) had contracted SARS, and five had died.

At that time, Hong Kong was hardly aware of the looming epidemic. Yet it was apparent to most that as an economic and cultural hub in the region, and sharing a relatively permeable border with Guangdong,

Hong Kong might easily become a site of heavy contagion. On February 21, Dr Liu Jianglun, a nephrologist who had treated SARS patients in Guangzhou, came to Hong Kong for a banquet. He stayed at the Metropole Hotel. Via a spreading mechanism that still baffles experts,[1] other hotel guests contracted the disease and subsequently carried SARS to Vietnam, Canada, Germany, Singapore, and Ireland. Locally, a 26-year-old man who came to the Metropole to visit a friend also contracted the virus. He was later admitted to the Prince of Wales Hospital (PWH) and spread the infection to the staff and students there.[2]

On March 11, more than twenty health-care workers on ward 8A of PWH were showing symptoms of atypical pneumonia. Within the next few days, nearly a third of the medical staff in the Department of Medicine also showed symptoms. All the standard microbiological investigations were negative, and those involved remained baffled as to whether staff members had contracted a mutated virus, an obscure pathogen, or something entirely new. The infection continued to spread. Fears grew. Afraid that they might contract the virus in such a confined space, the staff of the eleven-story PWH ceased using the elevators, and the stairways of the building were crowded with panic-stricken health-care workers.[3] To improve the ventilation, most staff kept their windows opened. The parking spaces closest to the main building, which, of course, had previously been the most sought after, were suddenly stigmatized as staff sought to keep their automobiles as far from the building as possible.

Before long, many departments in the hospital and medical school decided to divide their staff into "dirty" and "clean" teams. The dirty team would enter the SARS wards to look after patients, whose numbers were escalating. Most patients were themselves health-care workers who had contracted the infection while caring for others. The clean team was barred from these wards. This was not simply in order to confine the infection, however. There was an unspoken sense that the clean team would be entrusted with "carrying on" or "ensuring the future" of the hospital should the dirty team perish. There was a genuine fear of dying; and indeed affected medical staff were extremely ill, some on respirators, and some would die.

Around the same time, the infection was also spreading to the community. One of the most severely affected places was the Amoy Gardens, a residential complex housing thousands. Block E was particularly hard hit. By March 31, 107 of 200 residents of the block were living with SARS. The government decided to quarantine the entire building complex. The lay public, just as confused as the experts and authorities, speculated about the causes and means by which the infection was spreading: cockroaches, rats, sewage pipes, elevator buttons, or construction workers urinating nearby the apartment complex. Until the Amoy Gardens outbreak, most local citizens believed that they could avoid SARS by not leaving their homes. But now the home itself had become a dangerous site. In response, most families started the ritual of cleaning the furniture and floor daily with diluted bleach solution. The acrid stink of chlorine bleach quickly became a regular reminder of the perils of daily life.

Another ritual that had become common was the "undressing procedure" on returning home. In an attempt to maintain a SARS-free personal space, most Hong Kongers developed series of rituals to which they adhered when they crossed from dirty public space into what they hoped was a clean personal and family environment (e.g., the inside of the car or home). In his correspondence during the outbreak, one of the authors of this chapter (DL) described his undressing ritual as follows:

> Returning home from outside is like trying to undress before entering a clean operation theater. First we left the shoes outdoors, then we sneaked in, and asked Carissa [DL's two-year-old daughter] to wait . . . rushed straight into the bedroom and got hold of the plastic bag that was left there intentionally in the morning. Then we would undress in slow motion so that the virus would not pass around, and we would put everything into the plastic bag. And then tie a

knot. And then we would have a bath, brushing the whole body thoroughly to make sure no germs would be left. And then put on clean clothing and carefully take the bag to the domestic helper who would leave it aside for 24 hours before opening it for washing. This is to make sure that any virus on the clothing would die before the bag is opened. Some of my friends would leave the bag for even 48 hours and change all clothing in the office before starting work and before returning home.

Before slipping into the car, I always wipe my hands with alcohol-soaked tissue paper and I repeat this before I get out. Many people continue to wear a mask even when alone in the car. You can imagine how cautious people are in public transport. In the MTR [mass transit system railway], if one person sneezes, all the people nearby would rush away, literally. . . .

Other rituals include wearing a mask in all public spaces. Only press the elevator buttons with your key—to avoid contaminating the fingers. Wipe all supermarket shopping [items] with diluted bleach before putting them into the refrigerator. And of course, all the magazines need the same treatment.

At first we did not eat out . . . but gradually we gave in. But we would pick restaurants that were dead quiet. All waiters wore surgical masks. And we always picked a cubicle so that we were protected. And we never touch the doors, we just kicked open the door, like surgeons do in the operating theatre. Only disposable chopsticks are used, and in many restaurants there are now alcohol machines that let you wash your hands before the meal. In Luk Yu,[4] the century-old ritual of giving you a packet of toothpicks (to show the waiter's approval of your presence) is now replaced by the ritual of giving you a packet of 70 percent alcohol-soaked tissue paper.

Fear peaked on April Fools' Day, when a 14-year-old boy hacked into the web site of *Mingpao*, a local newspaper well respected for its objective reporting, and posted a phony news story that Hong Kong would soon be declared an "infected port" and isolated from the world. By noon, the news had spread throughout the community. Thousands of people lined up in supermarkets to stock up on food and other basic necessities. The atmosphere was one of incipient panic; different events created mass hysteria.

On May 13, Dr. Joanna Tse Yuen-man—a young respiratory care resident—died after contracting SARS on the job. Dr Tse was the first doctor to die from SARS, and her death evoked public mourning and a profound outrage at the mistakes made by the government in its initial mismanagement of the SARS crisis. The government became the object of intense public criticism on radio programs, in newspaper editorials, and in Internet chat rooms. The anger and frustration cut across social divisions and, in fact, became something of a unifying force among the general population. Of course, there was also a popular search for heroes and acts of heroism amid the uncertainty. Ever since the 1997 handover, Hong Kong had been troubled by the specter of incompetent leadership more beholden to China's leaders in Beijing than to the citizens of Hong Kong. The SARS epidemic brought public distrust to new levels. Among the emerging heroes were Professor K. Y. Yuen, the microbiologist at Hong Kong University who first identified the SARS coronavirus, Professor Joseph Sung, who led the "dirty" team in looking after SARS patients at the Prince of Wales Hospital, and Professor Sydney Chung, dean of the Chinese University of Hong Kong Medical School, who contradicted the government by first revealing that the spread of SARS in the community was uncontrollable.[5] They were held in the highest regard. That they were elevated to the status of public heroes, if only temporarily, says a lot about what Hong Kong residents were desperately seeking as a moral response to feelings of uncertainty and contempt. They wanted a sense of courage in despair.

The Psychological Impact of the SARS Outbreak

A series of studies have been conducted examining the psychological impact of SARS on various segments of the population. Using different designs and methodologies, these studies attempted to map out how the general population, people who are at high risk, and SARS patients reacted to the epidemic. Studying the psychological impact of SARS was not easy. To begin with, it was challenging to maintain a composed orientation toward research amid the confusion of the outbreak, both for researchers and informants. The course of an epidemic is by definition unpredictable and spontaneous. In order to accommodate the sudden twists and turns of the course of illness, the studies needed to be designed and initiated within a short time frame. The overriding need to avoid spreading infection also called for creative methodological strategies. In some instances, where face-to-face interviews were necessary, researchers faced the risk of contracting the virus.

General Population

One of the most creative studies conducted during the SARS outbreak was the CLSA Face Mask Index. A finance firm surveyed the first 100 persons who passed by a fast food chain restaurant at Queensway[6] during the lunch hour. The survey started on April 11 and was carried on until May 16, covering the most frightening part of the epidemic. In doing so, the Index was able to map out the perceived risk posed by the outbreak among locals. According to the Index, residents' fear and anxiety peaked around April 22, when 71 percent of passers-by were wearing masks. Just two days before, China's health minister and the mayor of Beijing had been fired. The Chinese Ministry of Health also announced on the same day that there were 339 confirmed and 402 suspected cases of SARS in Beijing alone, nine times more than the previously released figures had indicated.

In another study, the psychological impact of SARS on the general population was examined in a telephone survey.[7] Between May 2 and 5, 2003, the Hong Kong Mood Disorders Center interviewed a random sample of 1,250 adults. They estimated that about 19 percent of the study population suffered from emotional disorders.[8] This was higher than in earlier surveys. Emotional disorders were more common among females (27 percent vs. 11 percent among males), especially housewives (29 percent), and people who worked in clerical, sales, and service capacities (22 percent). The study also found that respondents who had

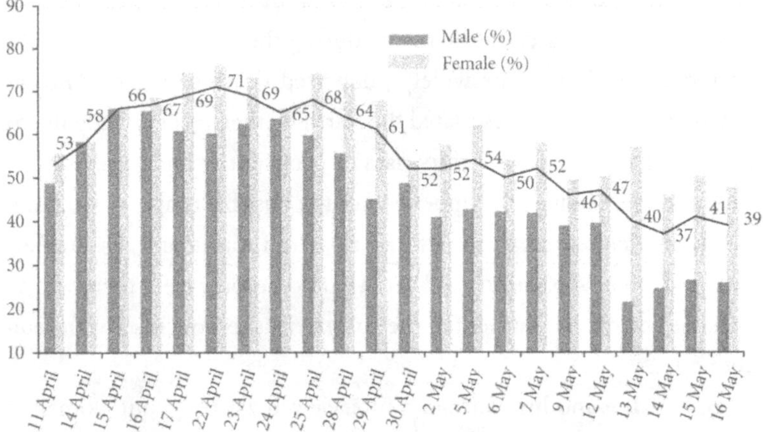

FIG. 7.1. CLSA HK Face Mask Index. Percent of first hundred people who pass by Delifrance at Queensway wearing a face mask after 1 P.M.

family members or workmates infected with SARS or who were aware of SARS infections in their residence or workplace were particularly stressed (25 percent vs. 17 percent of those who had not come into contact with SARS). The same study also found that two-thirds of the respondents constantly worried about themselves and their families contracting SARS. Nearly one-fifth of the respondents washed their hands more than fifteen times per day. Nervousness, inability to relax, frequent dreams, and impaired concentration were the symptoms most commonly reported by those who were distressed by the SARS outbreak.

The SARS Scare Among Pregnant Women

Pregnant women were particularly affected by the SARS epidemic. This was because ribavirin, the antiviral medication commonly used in SARS treatment, had documented teratogenicity in animals. Hence, if a pregnant mother became infected with SARS, she would face the dilemma of having to choose between rejecting ribavirin treatment or accepting its potential teratogenic effects on the fetus. This conundrum was heatedly discussed in the media during the SARS crisis, especially on radio talk shows. The widely publicized death of three SARS-infected pregnant women escalated the alarm further. Hence, studying the emotional and behavioral responses of pregnant women provided us with a means to gauge the upper end of the possible range of reactions. (Sadly, it later became apparent that ribaviran was in any case ineffective against the SARS agent; indeed, it would become clear there was no effective anti-viral treatment of the coronavirus responsible for the epidemic.)

D. T. S. Lee and his colleagues interviewed 235 pregnant women in April and May 2003 and compared them with 939 women interviewed before the SARS outbreak.[9] About one-fifth of the pregnant women believed that it was likely that they or their newborns might contract SARS. An equal number of participants worried about their older children contracting SARS at school or on their way to school.

As a result, 37 percent of the women did not go outside or did so only rarely. Another 55 percent avoided going out as far as possible. Eight percent of the women wore face masks all the time, while 63 percent wore masks regularly. A total of 40 percent of the participants washed their hands substantially more frequently than before. Another 52 percent washed their hands a little more frequently than before.

Stress, unhappiness, irritability, anxiety, fear, and a sense of helplessness were commonly experienced by these women. Between 7 percent and 10 percent of the women reported being substantially more affected by these emotions than before. Between 52 percent and 64 percent rated themselves more affected by these emotions than before.

SARS Patients

SARS infection and its treatment are a tremendous strain on the affected patients. In the most extreme cases, patients became psychotic. During the SARS outbreak, we noticed that a small but worrying number of patients developed disturbing psychotic symptoms and behavior. The occurrence of psychosis among SARS patients posed a profound challenge and threat to the clinical team. This is because patients with SARS-related psychosis, influenced by the elation, irritable mood, hallucinations, delusions, agitation, and hyperactivity, are unlikely to comply with clinical management and infection-control guidelines. In the extreme case, when a psychotic state jeopardized the safety of the patients or clinical staff, involuntary restraint and sedation became unavoidable. Yet, even with protective apparel, the clinical team still faced a substantial risk of contracting SARS in the course of their work, and their risk of infection was compounded by psychological dilemmas.

In examining the occurrence and risk factors of SARS-related psychosis, the liaison psychiatrists in Hong Kong found that about 1 percent of SARS patients were so troubled by psychotic complications that psychiatric consultations were sought.[10] Among them, the most likely clinical diagnosis was steroid-induced mania or psychosis. Family psychiatric history (33 percent v. 0 percent, c2 =11.3, df=1, p=0.002) was significantly more common among SARS patients with psychosis. There was also a higher rate of family member(s) contracting SARS among psychotic SARS patients (40 percent v. 13 percent), but the trend was not statistically significant (c2 =4.11, df=1, p=0.06). The SARS psychosis patients received significantly higher cumulative doses of steroids during their inpatient stay than the controls (10975mg v. 6780mg hydrocortisone equivalent; mw=125.5, df=43, p=0.017). The mean daily steroid dose for the SARS psychosis cohort was also higher than that of the controls, but the trend was not statistically significant (568mg v. 482mg hydrocortisone equivalent per day; mw=164, df=43, p=0.142). It thus appears that SARS-related psychosis is not a simple direct steroid toxicity. Rather, it is the combined result of steroid psychotogenic effects with personal vulnerability and possibly concurrent psychosocial stressors.

Post-SARS Psychiatric Morbidities

It is important to appreciate that steroid-induced psychosis is not the only psychiatric complication of SARS. A wide spectrum of psychiatric disorders was found during the acute and convalescence phase of the illness. One of the authors of this chapter (YKW) and his colleagues examined 134 SARS patients two to three weeks post-discharge.[11] Using a standardized diagnostic interview (Structured Clinical Interview for DSM-IV) and widely accepted diagnostic criteria (DSM), they found that 45 percent of the patients developed one or more forms of psychiatric disorders following SARS infection. About 13 percent of the patients suffered from organic mood disorders, 11 percent from major depression, 11 percent from adjustment disorders, 7 percent from post-traumatic stress disorder (PTSD), 5 percent from generalized anxiety disorders, and 2 percent from transient delirious or psychotic disorders. Patients who had been admitted to the Intensive Care Unit (OR 3.3, $p<0.05$) or had family members dying from SARS (OR 3.9, $p<0.05$) were more likely to have psychiatric complications.

More studies are needed to examine the longer-term psychological consequences of SARS. In particular, many survivors of SARS complained of profound lethargy and disturbing forgetfulness. Whether these disabling symptoms are due to the high-dose steroid treatment, as many patients believe, or are actually caused by undetected depression, sub-syndromal PTSD, or undetected SARS infection in the central nervous system awaits further investigation.[12]

Psycho-Political Responses

Most psychological studies of public trauma have focused on the negative impact of catastrophe. Notwithstanding the fact that traumatic events do take a heavy toll on the psychological well-being of those who are exposed, it is important not to forget that many people emerge from trauma stronger and more mature than before. In the participant observation and the ethnographic interviews, we encountered many individuals who were not only resilient to the overwhelming stresses associated with the SARS epidemic but had actually transcended the crisis and become psychologically stronger than before. If we may take this to a collective level, it would be legitimate to ask whether the SARS outbreak did any good to Hong Kong people generally and to the society as a whole.

One outcome of the consequences of the SARS outbreak was a demonstration on July 1, 2003, the sixth anniversary of Hong Kong returning to China. Attended by half a million Hong Kong citizens, the demonstration was only second in size to the demonstrations in 1989 that protested the Tiananmen massacre. Demonstration on such a scale is highly unusual, as there has not been a culture of demonstration in Hong Kong. If anything, Hong Kongers are better known for their political coolness. Freedom of speech and demonstration have not been impaired since the 1997 transition. Yet, despite profound economic and social hardship, until the July 1 demonstration, nearly all post-1997 demonstrations were on the scale of a mere few hundred people, if not a few dozen.

So what contributed to the July 1 demonstration? Was there a yearning for democracy? The July 1 demonstration was essentially construed in such a way by the Western media, who saw it as a cry for democracy. Notwithstanding that the demonstration itself was precipitated by a political crisis related to a controversial anti-subversion bill, the forces driving the half million demonstrators were more complex. An examination of the banners displayed in the demonstration quickly confirms the centrality of the anti-subversion Act 23. Yet also prominent among the banners were messages of discontent with the Tung administration, including dissatisfaction over how the SARS crisis was managed. One banner called for an independent enquiry into the SARS crisis, and another asked for the government's accountability for the 297 persons who

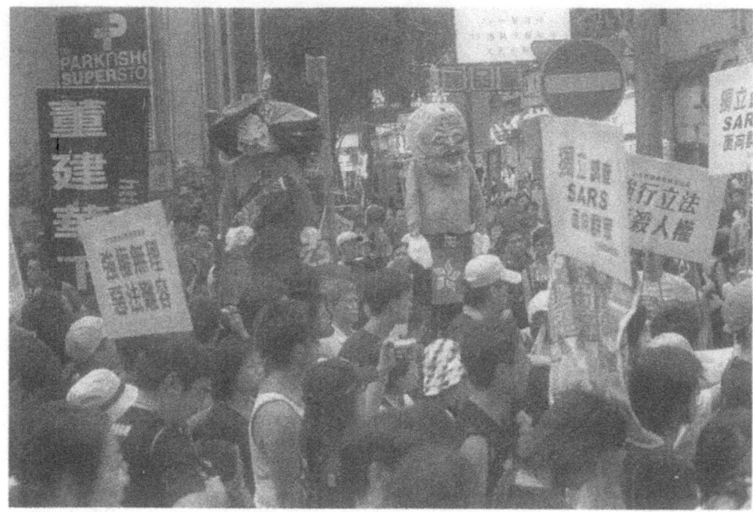

FIG. 7.2. Hong Kong demonstration of July 1, 2003. Photograph courtesy of *Apple Daily*, Hong Kong.

had died from SARS.[13] Black masks were worn by another cohort to express their dissent.

Would there have been a demonstration on July 1 had there not been a SARS outbreak? The replies we gathered from informants were unanimously negative. Indeed, two subsequent demonstrations, one against the anti-subversion legislation and another one against Tung himself, were poorly attended by local citizens. It would be incorrect to suggest that the July 1 demonstration was chiefly caused by the SARS outbreak, but without the epidemic, it would have been hard to mobilize half a million Hong Kongers on the street. Even the secretary of security, Regina Yip, acknowledged that not all the participants on July 1 were protesting the anti-subversion act. Some participants, she pointed out, had joined the demonstration to protest the incompetent management of the SARS outbreak.[14]

As M. E. DeGolyer justly pointed out, "The massive protest on 1 July also had roots in an unenviable record of mistakes and bad luck on the part of the Tung administration. However, the three most immediate contributors were the controversy over Article 23, the mishandling of SARS and the perceived failure of the new 'accountability system' to deliver the promised accountability and improvement in performance. The factors proved to be mutually reinforcing."[15] DeGolyer's view was closely echoed in the reflections written down by citizens on a July 1 demonstration advertisement board in Mong Kok—unnecessary SARS deaths as a result of incompetent administration were listed as one of the top reasons for attending the demonstration.

Unlike most major demonstrations, which took place amid discontent and dissatisfaction, the July 1 demonstration was not associated with a single incident of disorder or unrest. Even the commissioner of police praised the participants for their model behavior. Peaceful demonstrations on such scale are hard to find in the history of Hong Kong. Had the outbreak forced Hong Kongers to mature? Had the disease forced individuals to reassess their personal priorities? Had the crisis helped society to establish a solidarity that had been so lacking after the 1997 transition? What will be the long-term impact of SARS on the psycho-politics of postcolonial Hong Kong? These are questions with no simple answers. But perhaps history will tell whether the SARS outbreak has had any long-lasting positive effects on the psychology and politics of Hong Kong society.

CHAPTER EIGHT

Making Light of the Dark Side

SARS Jokes and Humor in China

HONG ZHANG

On May 16, 2003, a news article with the catchy title "Flirting with SARS and Seeking Pleasure from Suffering" appeared in a mainstream Chinese newspaper, *Beijing Qingnian Bao* (Beijing Youth Daily). Its author, Jiang Yu, wrote:

> Since April, people's life in Beijing has been dominated by "SARS." People listen to SARS news when at work and talk about SARS when they are off work. The media broadcast SARS news nonstop. . . . SARS even haunts people in their sleep and gives them nightmares. . . . However, although they are tortured by SARS physically, people in Beijing have not abandoned their optimistic outlook on life and their love for humor. On the contrary, at the spiritual level, people in Beijing courageously choose to crack jokes about SARS.[1]

SARS (severe acute respiratory syndrome), a deadly new infectious disease, wreaked havoc in China's capital city from mid April to mid May of 2003. In addition to producing fear among the populace, it also resulted in drastic changes in people's lives. Schools were closed, streets deserted, restaurants and shopping centers abandoned, weddings postponed, lovers and family members separated. Certain parts of the city were under quarantine, and people retreated into their homes for fear of catching the disease. Although Beijing residents were living with the threat of contracting SARS and had to endure major disruptions in their daily lives, they rose to the occasion with an outpouring of SARS jokes. SARS was even renamed "Smile and Retain Smile."[2] On the face of it, SARS jokes are about SARS, but they go far beyond that. Some jokes are political satires, while others poke fun at fears of, and panic reactions to, SARS. Thanks to the Internet and mobile phones, these jokes spread far and wide, spontaneously forming a kind of SARS subculture. In addition to revealing the Chinese people's views on the SARS outbreak, the jokes also reveal a host of other interpersonal, social and political problems in contemporary Chinese society.

In this chapter, I briefly describe some SARS jokes in order to explore their social and psychological implications. Most of the jokes were collected from various Internet web sites, where they were posted in an anthology format under such headings as "SARS Humor" ("Feidian youmou"), "A Complete Anthology of SARS Humor" ("Feidian youmou daquan"), "SARS Jokes" ("Feidian xiaohua"), and so on.[3] Altogether, more than 150 items were collected. This is by no means a complete list, because it is likely that some jokes were omitted from collected anthologies. Items were dispersed in hundreds, perhaps thousands of personal web sites, and those that circulated orally but were not recorded are missing from this study. However, jokes that appeared in Internet collections were probably better known to more people and were also more frequently and widely circulated. Therefore, a study of these more broadly circulated jokes can give us a general indication of their content and what sentiments they revealed.

This chapter is divided into two parts. In the first part, I categorize SARS jokes into six groups on the basis of the content. In the second, I present interpretations of the social implications of SARS jokes. I must also point out that it is impossible to include all the SARS jokes for analysis here, because there are not only a large number of them, but they also vary greatly in genre, style, and content. The term "joke" is also broadly defined here, since the humor in many SARS jokes does not lie in a particular witty punchline but is created through rhyming, word-play, parallel structure, punning, parody, personification, mockery, and mock advertisements. We must also bear in mind that many SARS jokes defy translation, because their comic effect derives from the rhymes and parallelisms in a way that is unique to the monosyllabic and tonal nature of the Chinese language.

1. Categories of SARS Jokes

SARS Jokes as Political Satire

It is generally believed that in societies living under repressive regimes, subversive political jokes often serve as a safety valve for people to voice their grievances and dissatisfaction with the status quo. In China, however, under the tight political control of the Mao era, there was very little room for political satire. Commenting on the muted nature of public political satire during the repressive years under Mao, Perry Link and Kate Zhou note: "The cataclysmic events of the Mao era produced dissatisfaction, but through the same years, repression was sufficiently strong, and penalties sufficiently severe, that a public or even semi-public *shunkouliu* (satirical slippery jingle) subculture could not develop."[4] In the relatively more open political atmosphere of the reform era of the past two decades, one prominent new social phenomenon in China is that political satires and subversive jokes have surfaced with vigor. They may not appear in the official press or mainstream media, but they are openly and eagerly exchanged at casual social gatherings by word of mouth, and more recently via Internet and mobile phone messages.[5] Most often, these political satires chastise official corruption, hypocrisy, and bureaucratic inefficiency, but some also target individual political leaders. Xu Yufang reported in 2002 that many political jokes mocking Jiang Zemin's "Three Represents" were circulated throughout China's capital city. Yu cited one as follows:

China and Russia finally agreed to do away with Iraq's Saddam Hussein. George W. Bush was jubilant and bought Vladimir Putin and Jiang Zemin a drink.

"Tomorrow I will deploy three B-2 bombers to blow Saddam's house to rubble, then he'll surely die," confided Bush.

"That is not 100 percent sure," commented Putin. "Let me deploy three Russian blondes and they will certainly exhaust the man to death," volunteered the former spy in a fashion compatible with his background.

"Still not good enough," said Jiang. "My method is most perfect." Then the 76-year-old statesman showed off his talent. "I need only to deploy my 'Three Represents' and they will surely bore him to death."[6]

Jiang's "Three Represents" has been hailed by the party propaganda machine as his breakthrough contribution to communist theories. Before he stepped down in November 2002 from the post of party chief, Jiang managed to have his "Three Represents" theory written into the Communist Party's bylaws, in an attempt to put himself among the ranks of communist icons such as Marx, Lenin, Stalin, Mao, and Deng. To the general public, however, Jiang's "Three Represents" theory was no more than boring political jargon, an inspiration only for making jokes. With the SARS outbreak, Jiang's "Three Represents" was "hijacked" by a hilarious SARS's version of "Three Represents" (the highlighted words are those rephrased from Jiang's Three Represents)[7]:

SARS's "Three Represents":

It represents the development trend of *viruses of a special kind.*

It represents the orientation of a *terror* culture.

It represents the fundamental interests of the overwhelming majority of *wild animals.*

One frequent theme in China's political jokes in the 1990s concerns the legacy that each of China's paramount leaders has left the people. A few years ago, a popular ditty read like this:

When Chairman Mao waved his hand, the whole nation went to the countryside [*xia xiang*].

When Deng Xiaoping waved his hand, the whole nation "jumped into the sea" [*xia hai*].

When Jiang Zemin waved his hand, the whole nation was laid off [*xia gang*].

The SARS virus struck China at a time when political leadership in China had just devolved to a new and younger generation—representing the most sweeping change in power since the death of Mao in 1976. The new government of President Hu Jintao and Premier Wen Jiabao promised new reform initiatives, and prior to the SARS outbreak, China's economy was robust and hopes were riding high that the country's new leaders would lead it to greater prosperity. When the SARS virus gave the whole nation and its new leaders a jolt, Chinese people responded by drawing on the epidemic to construct a new legacy concerning their leaders past and present. One SARS joke, titled "Follow Our Masters," says:

Following Old Mao, we mastered slogan-shouting,
Following Old Deng, we mastered cash-counting,
Following Old Jiang, we mastered stock-speculating,
Following Little Hu, we mastered face-mask-wearing.

The humor in this piece derives from the perfect rhyming, and the witty but nonetheless accurate characterization of China's leaders. Although there is a cynical tone conveyed, the subversive element is rather mild.

However, there is no ambiguity in this SARS-inspired joke, which explicitly takes the Chinese Communist Party to task:

What the Party Has Failed to Do, SARS Has Succeeded in Doing

The party failed to control dining extravagantly. SARS did.

The party failed to control touring with public money. SARS did.

The party failed to control having a sea of meetings. SARS did.

The party failed to control deceiving one's superiors and deluding one's subordinates. SARS did.

The party failed to control prostitution and whoring. SARS did.

What makes this SARS joke particularly poignant and cutting to the quick is the sarcastic irony that although we may have no cure for SARS, it can itself remedy the failures of the party to correct social ills, many of which are the party's own creations.

Jokes Depicting Panic Reactions to SARS

Although some SARS jokes were created to make a political statement, the majority comment on the panic reactions caused by the fear of SARS. Although much of the panic was due to the fact that SARS was a new and highly contagious disease with no known cure, the government's failure to take prompt action during the early stages of the SARS outbreak was also to blame. The SARS virus originally emerged in Guangdong, in southern China. For fear of criticism from Beijing and negative publicity abroad, local officials in Guangdong banned media reports about the disease. By mid March 2003, SARS had made inroads into twenty-six countries, becoming a global public health threat. Even as the disease began to spread in Beijing's hospitals in early April, officials there took no specific action and continued to claim that the SARS epidemic was under control. As a result, many people in the capital city of about 14 million continued to think that SARS was a "strange disease" that was restricted to a far-off province and that therefore it was of minor significance to them. But on April 20, 2003, the Chinese government suddenly reversed course by admitting to a nearly tenfold spike in SARS cases in Beijing and began to take drastic measures against SARS, calling on the nation to wage a "people's war" against it. Although the government's switch to candor and accountability demonstrated the leadership's new resolve to deal with the SARS outbreak transparently, instead of seeking to calm the public, the policy reversal and the daily triple-digit jump in SARS cases sparked widespread panic among Beijing residents. In a matter of days, the atmosphere in Beijing transformed from unease to panic as fear and anxiety gripped the populace.

One SARS joke offers a vivid description of how Beijing residents were trying to come to grips with their phobia about SARS and with the sudden changes in their lifestyles:

Beijing's "Four More"

> More people are drinking herbal medicine than morning tea.
> More people are quarantined for having a fever than for having complaints.
> More people are breaking out in a cold sweat at the sound of a cough or sneeze than when they are robbed.
> More people are wearing face masks than are wearing breast masks [bras].

Fear of long-term quarantine sent Beijing residents into panic purchasing of basic foodstuffs. Face masks, disinfectant, and Chinese herbal medicines were considered the latest "must have" preventive items, and were sold out the moment new shipments arrived. Some SARS jokes that began to circulate depicted SARS phobia as a "new disease"—"SARS phobia syndrome" (*feidian kongju zheng*), and one joke summarizes its "symptoms" as such:

> News flash, the cases of SARS phobia syndrome in our city have now reached 2.5 million. The specific symptoms of SARS phobia syndrome are:
> Take medicines indiscriminately and wear face masks
> Eyebrows are narrowed (due to worry), and unable to laugh
> Rush to buy cooking oil, rice, and Chinese herbal medicine
> Disinfect day and night without [getting] any sleep

In the midst of the SARS phobia, heightened by the government's stringent quarantine measures, a simple cough, a small sneeze, or a slight elevation of body temperature became equivalent to SARS symptoms and could be enough to subject one to mandatory quarantine or isolation. The uncertainty and the fear about SARS gave rise to stigmatization. Not only SARS patients, but the patients' friends and relatives, and even medical workers treating SARS patients were shunned by other people. Fear and anxiety also led to overreaction out of self-protection. There were reports that fires resulted from people putting their face masks, mobile phones, and money into microwaves for sterilization. Some SARS jokes began to use such titles as "How Does a Normal Person Die of SARS?" or "Several Ways of Dying from SARS" to remind the panicky public that prejudices, ignorance, and fear can be more "deadly" than the SARS virus itself. The following is one called "Ten Ways of Dying from SARS" ("Feidian de shizhong sifa"):

1. Being poisoned to death by an overdose of Chinese herbal medicine
2. Burned to death from a fire caused by boiling vinegar [a folk remedy]
3. Stifled to death by wearing face masks all the time
4. Scared to death after learning that your co-workers have SARS
5. Chopped to death by friends and relatives after coming back from a SARS-infected area
6. Cursed to death for spreading rumors through the Internet
7. Trampled to death for sneezing in a public place
8. Walked to death as a result of going on foot to one's workplace for fear of taking public transportation
9. Depressed to death about being taken to a mental hospital (a result of worrying too much that one might be a suspected SARS case)
10. Finally, really contracting the SARS virus and dying from it

Through deliberate exaggeration, this SARS joke exposed the absurdities in the overblown SARS phobia. It is also interesting to note that many SARS jokes were not one-time products but were subject to expansion and mutation as new situations occurred or different individuals added their personal touches. This is especially true of SARS jokes that list "different ways of dying from SARS." I found at least six different versions touching upon this theme on multiple web sites. While these "death" lists chronicled the mounting frenzied reactions to the SARS outbreak as a traumatized public was overwhelmed by fear of SARS, they also served as a scathing criticism of the prejudices and ignorance resulting from the SARS phobia.

Jokes Playing on the Government's Efforts to Control SARS

The government's declaration of war on SARS and its mass mobilization campaign also inspired some jokes that, on the face of it, resonate with the government's warlike rhetoric. When you are in a war, you need warriors, soldiers, and brave people who are willing to be martyrs. The official media repeatedly invoked words such as "warriors" (*zhanshi*), "brave person" (*yongshi*), and "martyr" (*lieshi*) to extol people fighting on the front line against SARS. Medical workers who died or fell sick when treating SARS patients were eulogized as heroes who were sacrificing their lives for a heroic cause. This joke talks about "warriors," "bravery" and "martyrs," but with a new twist:

> If you still go to work, you are a warrior.
> If you still dare to roam around on the streets, you are a brave person.
> If you are not replying to the messages I just sent you, you are a martyr.
> If you still insist on treating me to a dinner, well, then, I say you are a gentleman.

With China bracing for a crisis and the government calling for the whole nation to battle for a common cause, the national anthem seemed the most befitting and effective means to inspire patriotism. More than seven decades ago, the song "March of the Volunteers" inspired millions of Chinese people to rise up against the Japanese invaders.[8] In the battle against SARS, the government media accordingly used new campaign slogans adapted from the Chinese national anthem: "Millions of hearts with one mind battle against SARS" ("Wanzhong yixin, kangji feidian"), "The will of the masses will form a Great Wall for SARS prevention" ("Zhongzhi chengcheng, yufang feidian"). Soon, however, alternative SARS versions of the Chinese national anthem came into being:

> Arise,
> Ye who refuse to be *infected,*
> With our *money,*
> Let us build our Great Wall *against SARS*!
> The peoples of China are in the most critical time,
> Everybody must roar his defiance.

Seal off the doors!
Seal off the buildings!
Seal off the city!

Another SARS version of the national anthem had a slightly different ending. Instead of playing on the theme of quarantine measures, it asks for "material" compensation:

Arise,
Ye who refuse to be *infected,*
With our *money,*
Let us build our Great Wall *against SARS*!
The peoples of China are in the most critical time,
Everybody must roar his defiance.
Give us money.
Give us medicines.
Give us face masks.

In order to mobilize the masses for the fight against SARS, the government repackaged Mao-era rhetoric to rally the nation for a patriotic "people's war." The state-run news media, while showing some signs of more openness and freedom in reporting on SARS, were also devoted to portraying a society unified in a heroic fight. But one SARS joke shows a somewhat different picture by indicating that different sectors of the society responded to SARS with their own agendas:

The government's declaration: war on SARS
The media's front page: [news] about SARS
Experts' suggestions: prevention of SARS
Drugstores sell medicine: in the name of SARS
Friends meet, trading information on SARS
A co-worker coughs, a frightful cry—"SARS!"

The government's adoption of a Mao-style political campaign to combat SARS inspired mock Mao poems. By cleverly altering a few words and lines, these hilarious jokes appeared as new SARS poems in

"Maoist" disguise. Mao was well known for his ability to write elegant poems in classical style, and imitating his poems was no small feat. Daring to rewrite and play on Mao poems thus became an opportunity to show off both one's ingenuity and one's defiance of authority.

SARS Phobia Transformed into Comic Moments of Laughter

The humor in some SARS jokes lies in their dark comedy or bitter sarcasm, but in others, the effect is comic and funny. Wearing a face mask showed that people were apprehensive, but numerous SARS jokes found humor in face-mask-wearing. In a sweet and playful tone, one said:

> Wearing no face mask accentuates the beauty of your face,
> Wearing a face mask highlights the beauty of your eyebrows,
> With or without a face mask, you are beautiful in my mind.

Using the elements of surprise and personification, another SARS joke makes face-mask-wearing a moment of sensuous pleasure:

> Gently brush your hair behind your ears.
> Tenderly caress your face.
> Sweetly kiss your lips.
> Gotcha! I am a face mask, remember to wear me!

Mixing self-pity with quixotic passion, one lost lover cleverly pokes fun at himself while also making fun of the quarantine measures:

> I wrote your name in the sky, but the wind took it away.
> I wrote your name on the sand, but a wave took it away.
> I was busy worrying about you and let out a few dry coughs; the SARS-prevention group took me away.

Through self-mockery, one individual made the following "confession": "Last night I had a dream in which I encountered a beautiful woman. Consequently, I developed preliminary SARS symptoms: high fever, difficulty in breathing, and dry coughs with blood [actually, nose bleeding].” Some SARS jokes were a hybrid of mixed messages. They were half-joking and half-serious, creating a comic effect by making multiple comments on the battle against SARS but not taking a particular stand. Imitating the classical poem “Haoliao ge” (“The Done Character Song”), each line of which ends with the character *liao*,[9] a SARS version of “The Done Character Song” (“Liao zi ge”) came into being:

> Guangdong was first stricken with SARS, then Beijing got infected.
> The government relaxed its control, so the media dare to make a fuss now.
> Many people have contracted SARS, and the hospitals are full.
> Medical workers have got rough jobs; they are risking their lives on the front line.
> The masses are out of their wits; they wear face masks to cover their faces.
> The WHO is now in charge; full containment is not far off.
> Get your three doses of herbal medicine prepared and go and get some exercise.

Done in the form of a child’s nursery rhyme, some SARS jokes also use advice about SARS prevention to warn their lovers against something else:

> My sweetheart [husband/boyfriend/lover], you go to work,
> Make sure you wear your face mask tight.
> Climb the stairs [i.e., avoid the crowd in the elevator].
> Eat instant noodles for lunch.
> Look straight ahead,
> Eyesight can also be contagious.
> Don’t hold the hand of another girl,
> Your days will be numbered when I learn about it.
>
> The virus is spreading rapidly,
> Affecting everyone’s mood badly.
> I am worried that you may get infected,
> So I suggest that you not look too slick.
> Keep your distance when you speak,

> Get out quick in a crowded place.
> Wear a face mask when you go out,
> Cover up with a quilt when you go to sleep.
> Maintain a cheerful spirit,
> Give fewer kisses, eat more dishes.

In some SARS jokes, punning is used to create comic effects. Punning can make almost any situation comical by interpreting the situation in several different ways at the same time. The Chinese term for SARS is *feidianxing feiyan* (atypical pneumonia), *feidian* for short. Thus, in Chinese, "Wo feidian" conveys the dreadful confession "I have SARS." In other contexts, however, "Wo feidian" has a host of other meanings that are not even remotely related to SARS. This joke uses punning:

> Last Sunday, you came to my house and noticed that I had a string of firecrackers. You insisted on setting them off. I told you not to do so, because there was no holiday [to justify] the festivity. But you did not listen to me. With one hand holding a lighted cigarette butt and the other grabbing the firecrackers from me, you shouted at me: "For so many years, I have not had a chance to set firecrackers off. You are not going to stop me now. *Wo feidian. Wo feidian*!" All of sudden, three people with face masks broke into my house and took you away.

Here "Wo feidian" simply means, "I dare to set the firecrackers off." Interpreted out of context, however, it means, "I have SARS." The humor lies in the wrong interpretation taking precedence over the true meaning. Indirectly, this joke could be seen as poking fun at the government's massive quarantine measures, which may have been too drastically implemented. Apparently, this punning on "Wo feidian" was extremely popular among people who shared SARS jokes. According to one source, the "Wo feidian" joke above was forwarded 1.7 million times over the Internet.[10] There were at least thirteen different versions of SARS jokes playing on this same punning, including one that even made reference to the ongoing Iraq War and the antagonism between

Saddam Hussein and George W. Bush:

Saddam was found. Bush warned him not to set Iraq's oil wells on fire. Defying Bush's order, Saddam shouted: "Wo feidian. Wo feidian." Saddam was immediately taken to Beijing's Xiao Tangshan Hospital.[11]

Even Saddam was not spared being quarantined even though his "Wo feidian" really meant, "I dare to set the oil wells on fire."

Another joke describes an old lady's perplexity at the sudden big fuss over *feidian*. So she murmurs to herself: "If everyone is so afraid of *feidian*, then don't turn on the light." The pun lies in another interpretation of *feidian*: "costs too much electricity." Hence the old lady offered her simple "solution" to the problem—"Don't turn on the light."

SARS Jokes as Mock Directives, Advice, and Advertisements

As a new, hitherto unknown disease, SARS fed everyone's imagination as to how to protect themselves from it. Many jokes made the rounds as mock prevention advice. One such joke was labeled the "highest directive" (*zuigao zhishi*) in the Maoist style of the Cultural Revolutionary era:

The Highest Directive:
Wash your hands before meals and after shitting;
Wash your hands when going out and coming home;
Wash your hands after riding in a vehicle;
Wash your hands after you touch anything.

After the Chinese government reversed course and began to cooperate closely with the World Health Organization, which played a prominent role in coordinating the global response to SARS, "WHO" almost became a household word in China. Thus some jokes assume the form of WHO warnings. One of these ran: "According to the latest announcement made by the WHO, wearing a face mask cannot provide full protection against SARS. Because your lungs are located in your chest, wearing a bra is therefore a must. Everyone, men and women, must be sure to wear both a double-layered face mask and a double-layered bra when going out."

Some SARS jokes claimed that they were "folk prescriptions" (*pianfang*) or "secret remedies" (*mifang*) that had special SARS-prevention effects. One "folk prescription," in the style of concocted Chinese herbal medicine, tells people how to create "an effective quarantine" for oneself: "Mix garlic with stinking tofu in warm water, take half of the mixture orally and smear the other half on both cheeks in order to create a permanent 10-square-meter quarantine zone against the contraction of SARS."

The onslaught of SARS revealed the neglected state of China's public health-care system. Privatization has sent medical costs skyrocketing, leaving rural health care in a shambles. While laid-off urban workers saw their health-care benefits reduced, millions of rural migrant working in the cities did not have any health insurance at all and could not afford to seek medical care. In a desperate attempt to prevent the SARS epidemic from spreading into China's vast poor rural areas, the Chinese government ordered free medical treatment for all low-income urban and rural SARS patients who could not pay. However, there is an irony in the government's offer of free SARS treatment. In the freewheeling, money-driven economy created by the past two decades of reforms, anything like a "free ride" coming from the state sounds almost too good to be true. Tapping into this irony, one SARS joke turns the government's free medical treatment for SARS patients into a mock travel agency advertisement urging consumers to take advantage of "a free vacation package":

> My dear friends, want a vacation? To enjoy a supervalue complimentary seven-day stay in a hospital, inclusive of room and board, please dial the toll-free number 120 [the equivalent of 911 in the United States] without delay! If you call now, you will also get a free face mask, a stylish disinfected suit, and free pickup by ambulance. The first ten callers will also get free quarantine (private room service) treatment. Call now and mention the secret password: "I have a fever."

Jokes about the "Positive Impact" of the SARS Outbreak

Humor, as one type of self-reflective activity, can reveal unexpected perspectives and open up an alternative view of our world to us. After playing down the outbreak of SARS for months as no cause for concern, the Chinese government declared "a people's war" against the disease. The SARS virus was now the archenemy, because it had already created a health crisis in China, and might lead to huge economic fallout and widespread social instability. But in some SARS jokes that circulated over the Internet and mobile phones, the SARS crisis was portrayed as "benefiting" the Chinese people and Chinese society. Written in free-style verse, one SARS joke claimed that SARS has taught us some important lessons about life:

> It is through encountering SARS that we learn the true value of being able to breathe freely.
> It is by wearing face masks that we realize the importance of seeing the true face.
> It is during the times of great calamity that we find our friendship is truly valuable.

There are multiple implications in the above statements, because such expressions as "to breathe freely" (*ziyou huxi*) and to see the "true face" (*zhenshi miankong*) carry both literal and metaphorical meanings. They indirectly suggest that until confronted with the SARS crisis, the Chinese people had been living under deception and lies, and that, ironically, it was SARS that had made the truth come out and brought about new enlightenment. Some SARS jokes even had titles such as "On the Positive Aspects of SARS" ("Feidian de jiji yimian") or "Benefits Brought about by SARS" ("Feidian dailai de haochu"). In these jokes, rather than being perceived as "a menace" to society, SARS is embraced as "a blessing" because it has proved "effective" in everything from eradicating bad health habits to boosting nationalist spirits and improving social mores. Some "positive impacts" of SARS mentioned by these jokes were:

Everyone has begun to pay attention to personal hygiene now; the habit of washing hands has finally been fostered.
The status of traditional Chinese medicine has been enhanced, because overstocked herbal medicines were all sold out.
People have begun to respect one another's privacy now, because they dare not go out.
The street scenes of holding hands and kissing in public have been reduced; good social mores are thus facilitated.
The elderly and the disabled can have seats when riding the public buses now, because the buses are empty.
"Three-accompaniment girls" have no work now, so the moral standard of the society is improved.

It is not difficult to see the cynical message in these SARS benefits lists. Obviously, these SARS jokes were not about SARS per se but about social problems in China today. By focusing on the "positive impacts" of SARS in such a sarcastic way, the public vented their frustrations and criticisms of the party for its inability to resolve rampant social problems. It is interesting to note that, perhaps in the same spirit of casting SARS's "transforming" power in a positive light, one joke highlighted the "particular benefits" of the SARS crisis for married women—"Enumerating Several Major Benefits That SARS Has Brought to a Wife" ("Lishu 'feidian' gei qizi dailai de jida haochu"). The following is a brief summary:

The husband who normally does not wash his hands, feet, or take a shower will all of sudden wash his hands eight times a day and change his clothes daily.

The husband who never returns home before midnight all of a sudden becomes very homesick and quits his nightclubbing.

The husband who self-indulgently gorges on meat in restaurants all of a sudden turns into a rabbit and takes a fancy to the various vegetable dishes cooked at home, contending that eating vegetables may boost his immune system.

The husband who usually hates to walk all of a sudden puts on his sportswear and jogs every day. He now seems especially energetic to his wife.

The husband who always eyeballs every pretty woman in the street all of a sudden loses his target, because all he can see now is a square-shaped face mask.

This really makes his wife worry a whole lot less.

The husband who usually acts like a man of great importance all of a sudden becomes weak and feeble and asks his wife to check his forehead every ten minutes. That really makes his wife feel deeply appreciated.

It is not clear whether this joke appealed only to or was circulated among women. I found it in the Ana Club (Ana Julebu), an Internet chat room for women.[12] It was posted on April 28 and was accessed more than 6,147 times that same day. Over the next ten days or so, between April 28 and May 10, it was accessed at least 200,000 times. Some women also posted comments on this joke; some agreed with it and some did not. On the face of it, this joke may make one wonder what is going on with marital relations in China. However, perhaps more significantly, it is clear from this that women Internet users were frequently using online communication to reach out to one another and find a public forum to express their opinions in a way they might otherwise not have done.

2. The Social Significance of SARS Jokes

Why joke about something as serious as an outbreak of a deadly disease? What can SARS jokes tell us about China's fast-changing society and its people? At one level, finding humor in calamities is one way of dealing with fear and anxiety about the unknown. Writing on the perpetuation of AIDS jokes in the mid 1980s, Allen Dundes, an anthropologist and folklorist, says, "Disasters breed jokes." Sick jokes (jokes about a calamity or tragedy) "follow in the wake of horrible and tragic events" because "they constitute a kind of collective mental hygienic defense mechanism that allows people to cope with the most dire of disasters, natural or otherwise."[13] SARS was a life-threatening, highly contagious disease with the terrifying ability to spread in an uncontrollable way. The SARS virus certainly caused heart-wrenching fears and widespread panic among the public. Seeking humor in the midst of such fear and uncertainty can provide psychological relief and release by turning fear and anxiety into moments of laughter and comedy. As one SARS joke states: "In the days of the SARS epidemic, we do not have a vaccine, but we do have humor to keep us company." It was also a "safe" way to talk about the disease. People retreated from the streets, public entertainment, and meeting places, and discussing and exchanging SARS jokes was a way of continuing to socialize during dangerous times, a way of continuing to participate in a public life. Even if that public life was attenuated and suspended, there was still a virtual community of punsters, joke makers, web sites, and so on, available.

When discussing the existence of jokes of this kind, Dundes tends to emphasize that it is a universal phenomenon, "a natural psychic response to crisis." According to him, these jokes "would not come into existence if they did not answer some sort of deep psychological need." However, the outpouring of SARS jokes in China also indicates something more than just answering psychological needs. The very fact that these jokes appeared in large quantities, speaking with rich, diverse voices, suggests contemporary China's fast-changing political culture and society. In the past fifty years, there has been no lack of humanitarian calamities that frightened the public and took many lives in the People's Republic of China. However, the SARS jokes could have been possible in China only today, in the context of the rapid changes of the past two decades in economic and political conditions. On the one hand, there has been the emergence of a sizable and growing middle-class population whose economic independence makes them a force outside formal party and state structures; on the other hand, the emergence of a degree of government latitude allows the public to engage in different modes of expression and to voice social criticisms and dissatisfactions. Cracking jokes, in general, is very much in vogue as a form of popular culture in post-Mao China.[14] Being able to tell jokes has become associated with being cool, smart, rebellious, and independent—a way to demonstrate one's wit and cleverness with wordplay. Thus it was inevitable that practitioners would turn their attention to SARS when the SARS crisis became the dominant topic of the moment. The government's embarrassing cover-up, its sudden switch to candor and stringent control measures, and the public's panic reactions to this mysterious and potentially deadly disease all provided abundant materials for making jokes.

The range of SARS jokes was also quite varied. Some jokes were a kind of grass-roots commentary on the party's initial failure to respond to the crisis. They provided a context for people to share and discuss their anxieties and fears, to bond together and mitigate the seriousness of the situation. People spread information about SARS via mobile phones and the Internet, which were mostly outside of the government's control. Some criticized or made fun of the government. Others voiced people's frustration with the lack of information about the disease. Yet other people helped alleviate fear and anxiety through humor and laughter. Some used the jokes as commentaries on the Chinese character and social problems. Still others saw jokes as an opportunity to demonstrate their intellectual prowess, independence, and rebelliousness. The jokes were as varied in their construction and intent as the participants themselves, reflecting the concerns and, in some cases, the conceits of their progenitors.

There is no doubt that technological innovations in communication played a major role in the proliferation and variety of SARS jokes. Short and concise, SARS jokes circulated with a rapidity characteristic of the flows of goods and services in the information age, making their way from one user to another and then another. When concerned friends, colleagues, and family members sent each other the latest news on the SARS front over their mobile phones and through emails, they also passed on SARS jokes to raise morale. Very soon, a chain reaction of circulating and creating SARS jokes followed. Along the way, these jokes were commented on, added to, or even redone, with new material emerging in the process. Individuals, often faceless and identityless, delighted in their cleverness and inventiveness and competed with each other to the amusement of the virtual community of participants. To some extent, the SARS jokes themselves became "endemic" and "contagious," quickly transmitted by the Internet and mobile phones. As more SARS jokes spread and gained popularity, they fueled the public interest in creating even more. For an increasingly urban and more affluent Chinese population living in the information age and a global market economy, the Internet and mobile phones have created new public spaces where individuals find new outlets for displaying their creativity and individuality, as well as for expressing and sharing their emotions, fears, and opinions. This may partly explain why SARS jokes not only appeared in large quantity, but also varied greatly in content, genre, and style, ranging from emboldened political commentaries to playful self-mockery, from biting sarcasm to frivolous wordplay. In these newly created public spaces, the all-powerful state becomes less relevant and no longer dominates public discourse as it did in the past.

During the SARS outbreak in China, people were frightened and the whole nation was bracing for a crisis. Although belated, the government's new resolve to wage a "people's war" against the disease was vigorous and forceful. The battle against SARS was no laughing matter. To crack jokes at this heightened moment of national crisis seems at the very least out of tune with the party's call for national unity in the fight against SARS. However, so popular were these SARS jokes that even the government's own news services and sites began to collect and disseminate them.[15] On May 9, 2003, the party's Internet web site, Renminwang (www.people.com.cn), collected and published an anthology of SARS jokes under the title "Atypical Humor During the SARS Period" ("Feidian shiqi de feidianxing youmo").[16] Some of the jokes mentioned in this chapter were found on this web site. The editor's note for publishing these SARS jokes on Renminwang's web site included some revealing comments on the upsurge of SARS jokes:

> Perhaps it is because the Chinese people have gone through so much hardship and suffering that they have learned how to cope with a sudden and unexpected crisis. Although the SARS virus is still raging, our life is still going on as usual. Under the current conditions, when Internet and SMS [short messaging service] messages are in vogue, the Chinese people's wit and humor are given full play. It [telling SARS jokes] also demonstrates the Chinese people's optimistic view about life by seeking laughter in suffering. Let us read these concise, laughter-provoking messages and use laughter to face this "SARS time," which, we believe, will not last long.

To be sure, the party's web site did not dispense jokes that criticized the government—many politically sensitive jokes were omitted from Renminwang. However, the government did acknowledge both the positive dimension to keeping up humor in such times and the fact that SARS jokes and joking had captured the popular imagination in a way that could prove beneficial to its dealings with the crisis itself. Nonetheless, since these jokes were transmitted via communications networks that the government did not completely control, it also became necessary for the government to put on a "public face" as well. By allowing such materials to appear in official media, the government showed its own hand in this newly developing and expanding realm, making it seem more open, accepting, and accommodating.

The shift from the 1980s to the 1990s opened up new spaces for the transformation of public life and popular culture in China. In the 1980s, China was coping with the reversal of radical communism's ideas, programs, and institutions as it gradually opened its doors to the West. Fueled by unprecedented economic growth during the 1990s (which showered those living in urban China with newfound wealth and opportunities), China was catapulted full tilt into the frenetic assault of global capital, products, ideas, fashions, and trends. An ever-receding government gave way to an explosion of entrepreneurial activities and enterprises and the appearance of urban middle-class consumers who were ever more connected with one another and with the international community through global networks and channels. This connection was evidenced primarily in the exponential increase in the number of cell phones and Internet users.[17] This new class, well-educated, affluent, and in search of new forms of entertainment, leisure activities, and consumption, supplied the most fertile ground for the articulation, dissemination, and transformation of SARS jokes, the majority of which were exchanged via cell phone and Internet to an electronic community of users throughout China's cities. Judging from the dates when SARS jokes were posted on Internet web sites, it appears that most of them were created and circulated in late April and early May, coinciding with the height of the SARS crisis. SARS jokes had faded by the end of May, when the outbreak eased and life was beginning to return to normal. However, these jokes have left us with a unique legacy, providing us with a new lens through which to view a rapidly changing society and its spontaneous reactions to traumatic events.

Acknowledgment

I thank David Nugent and Constantine Hriskos for their comments on my earlier drafts of this chapter.

PART IV

Globalization and Cross-Cultural Issues

CHAPTER NINE

SARS and the Problem of Social Stigma

ARTHUR KLEINMAN AND SING LEE

Discrimination, negative labeling, menacing societal responses such as ostracism and exclusion, and even violence and suicide are characteristic of stigma.[1] These and other aspects of stigma were experienced by SARS patients and by others who are perceived to be potential spreaders of the epidemic (including family members, co-workers, neighbors, and health professionals), both inside China (including the Hong Kong Special Administrative Region, or HKSAR) and in Chinese communities outside China (e.g., in Singapore, Taiwan, Toronto, Canada, and the United States). Such stigma has been documented for earlier epidemics globally and for epidemics of plague, cholera, and smallpox in China.[2] It is also an aspect of China's current epidemic of HIV/AIDS. Albeit by no means identical, the stigmatization of SARS shares broad similarities with the stigmatization of other health conditions, including chronic disorders such as leprosy, HIV, epilepsy, and mental illness.[3] Yet stigma associated with the SARS epidemic of 2003 exhibits unique features, because the illness differs from other stigmatized conditions in crucial ways, such as its uncertain routes of transmission, the unusually vigorous surveillance and quarantine procedures needed, media-propelled fears of extreme contagiousness and high mortality, and the special vulnerability to it of health-care workers in large hospitals.[4]

Stigma matters, because it increases the suffering of affected individuals and their families, fosters noncompliance with treatment and other potentially dangerous responses, jeopardizes the relationship between health-care workers and patients, and undermines public health practices like early case identification and quarantine. It may also intensify "blaming the victim," scapegoating of marginal groups, negative mental health outcomes, and human rights abuses. In the workplace too, stigma can result in substantial management difficulties and consequent productivity loss.

Once it is unleashed, stigma is difficult to control and may injure individuals and groups. For example, despite efforts to educate the public on the nature of mental illnesses, psychiatric stigma remains rampant in all parts of the world.[5] In Chinese communities, where close social networks regulate individual behavior, and where advocacy and legal measures against discrimination are typically underdeveloped, stigma carries particularly powerful moral, emotional, and social consequences.

This chapter draws on available reports and research evidence on stigma connected with SARS and discusses its implications for social and public health, with a special focus on Chinese communities.

Reports of SARS-Related Stigma

In Hong Kong, stigmatizing practices related to SARS are reported to have penetrated almost all levels of everyday life. Some funeral homes refused to handle the bodies of SARS victims;[6] certain medical and paramedical staff were reluctant to care for SARS patients;[7] some SARS patients and their family members were shunned and forced out of employment.[8] Employees who had recently been to the hospital or to parts of mainland China where SARS was reported were asked to take annual leave.[9] Neighbors of two homes for the elderly in Shatin, HKSAR, demanded that all the windows of the homes be shut on the grounds that their inmates were vulnerable to SARS and would spread the virus to the community.[10] Many people who were not infected but residing in buildings associated with SARS were asked to take leave and refused basic services. Residents of Amoy Gardens, a residential complex with 17,000 inhabitants in nineteen blocks in the HKSAR, where a significant number of SARS cases occurred, were isolated in camps and shunned by co-workers and schoolmates, who would not share elevators or hallways with them. One man with SARS-like symptoms (i.e., sneezing) said that colleagues refused to use the same toilet or to eat with him.[11] Family members of SARS victims were kept away from the dead and dying, interfering with traditional mortuary rituals and with the process of bereavement.[12] Discrimination extended especially to health professionals, who were refused service at a barber shop, shunned by passengers on minibuses, and avoided by colleagues.[13] One woman was fired for refusing to promise not to see her boyfriend, who was, at the time, a nurse caring for SARS patients.[14] As of September 12, 2003, the Hong Kong Equal Opportunities Commission had received 80 complaints and 444 enquiries from people who had been treated for SARS, including recovered patients, about being shunned, ostracized, and isolated.[15]

Individual and Collective Experiences of SARS-Related Stigma

Often stigma operates along ethnic, racial, or gendered lines to disproportionately affect marginal groups. But in China, the stigmatization of SARS was not reducible to those categories of difference. In some instances, spatial divisions were key, most noticeably at Amoy Gardens.[16] "Why can't they send us to another site?" begged one resident. "They're basically telling us to wait here and die. We don't talk to our neighbors because everyone is afraid of contracting the disease from. . . . We're living in fear every day. [The workers here] leave the food outside the door and treat us as if we're lepers because they're afraid they'll get it too. They won't even speak to us."[17]

The litany of stigma experiences reported by residents of Amoy Gardens is overwhelming. Victoria Ng, a resident of the complex, was avoided by her brothers, sisters, and mother for over two months. The isolation was so painful that she "suffers bouts of sudden weeping and began taking antidepressants for the first time."[18] Ms. Cheung, a seven-year resident, was given a clean bill of health by her corporation's doctor, but she was nonetheless shunned by colleagues upon returning to the office. Other people living at Amoy Gardens reported feeling like fugitives. Block E was hit particularly hard. According to the HKSAR government's SARS expert committee, 41 percent of the 329 SARS infected cases in the Amoy Gardens were from Block E.[19] It is not surprising, then, that "Block E" or "Block E of the Amoy Gardens" became shorthand in Hong Kong for contagious individuals or groups and other vectors. Some residents were upset by the media's use of photos of the entranceway to Block E in metonymically referring to the outbreak in general. One uninfected resident of Block S said: "I felt so helpless that my business partners didn't want to meet me face to face. We couldn't do business as a result. Media-portrayed negative images about my identity as an Amoy Gardens resident were known as far as Hangzhou, China, and I had to pay a bribe in order to be offered a hotel room there. We were treated like monsters even outside of Hong Kong." Showing how deeply the fears associated with the stigma of SARS penetrated, impacting both the workplace and family life, he added: "My children became so fearful that they kept taking their own temperature. When they resumed classes, their classmates told them 'You were on the TV,' and my children quickly responded: 'I don't live in Block E.' "

In an ongoing study at Amoy Gardens, Sing Lee and his research staff at the Hong Kong Mood Disorders Center conducted two focus groups with fifteen residents in June 2003. The study found that even uninfected residents felt discriminated against in the workplace and at school and were shunned by service providers. Discrimination impacted the fabric of everyday life for many residents, determining or upsetting plans and introducing a patent sense of fear, even guilt, into social interactions. "I had a cold with coughs," said a 67-year-old uninfected resident of Block A, "and called to make an appointment with my general practitioner. But he was so afraid that he asked me not to go." A leader of the residents' association describes an environment of paranoia and social experiences akin to being outcast or exiled *within* society: "Amoy Gardens became a dead community, and it was frightening to walk [there] with no people around. Many people had moved out. The price of our flats dropped quickly by 15–20 percent." One Block E resident, although he had moved out of the housing complex prior to the outbreak, experienced mood disturbances upon returning there to pick up letters from the mailbox. Other residents were refused occupancy in hotels once their address was revealed.

Stigma and fear produced feelings of injustice and anger, but, just as forcefully, feelings of despair, loss of control, powerlessness. One Block E resident, an ex-SARS patient himself, who lost his wife to the outbreak, wept in the focus group: "My family, as ordinary citizens, had no choice but to send our dead ones to the crematorium. That was unfair. Why were they treated so differently from the deceased medical staff who were granted honorary funerals by the government? That is discrimination!"[20]

If spatial boundaries were central to processes of stigmatization, occupation was also a key factor, nurses and doctors becoming the primary victims of discrimination and shunning. That occupation alone served as a quilting point for popular fears and uncertainties is made evident by the fact that some nurses were forced to vacate their apartments even though the hospitals at which they worked did not treat SARS patients.[21] In a study of 1,271 health-care workers from a general hospital that was isolated because of a major SARS outbreak in southern Taiwan, M. Y. Chong found that psychiatric morbidity occurred in 75.3 percent of subjects. Feelings of extreme vulnerability, helplessness, and loss of control were common.[22] Ping-chung Leung of the Chinese University of Hong Kong accused the authorities of being "cold" to hospital staff and patients alike: "During the SARS outbreak . . . the authorit[ies] have overstressed scientific management and ignored the human touch between people . . . the authority's management has lacked sufficient care for its staff and their rights. We can see this in the number of cases in which nurses were crying out for protective gear."[23] Indeed, providing mental health services to vulnerable frontline workers was a challenge because of the additional stigma that is widely associated with seeking psychiatric treatment in China. Given the high prevalence of psychiatric morbidity among frontline health workers, however, lack of mental health intervention would not only compromise clinical care but also adversely affect their willingness to participate in clinical care in the future. Here, two modes of stigmatization converged onto a particular group of people to produce a dramatic, ongoing experience of social suffering, limiting efforts to seek help and possibilities for care or intervention.

Finally, stigma was particularly strong among ex-patients, who were routinely ostracized by communities and even by family members.[24] Extreme anger was expressed at so-called super spreaders ("kings of poison"), who were widely accused of being responsible for the epidemic.[25] In rural areas of mainland China, because accurate medical information was less accessible and because close social networks resisted bureaucratic intrusions, stigma could take on more brutal forms. In late April 2003, peasants blocked the construction of buildings geared to be hospitals for SARS patients, the first instance of civic violence directly associated with the disease. Partly built bedrooms were ripped apart, construction materials were burned, and the windows were shattered.[26] Other instances of violence quickly followed. In Beijing, fearful residents set up barricades on the outside of the city to try to keep out those traveling from SARS-affected areas. "We'll stay here and keep this roadblock," said one participant, "until the threat of SARS passes."[27] In Zhejiang province, angry villagers broke windows and furniture in a building where suspected SARS carriers were to be quarantined.[28]

A population-based survey in Hong Kong confirmed that stigmatizing attitudes and behaviors toward SARS were common, and these popular fears were directed primarily at ex-patients. A study carried out by the Hong Kong Mood Disorders Center as late as 3–8 July, 2003, found that over 70 percent of the 1,023 respondents in Hong Kong had been anxious about contracting SARS, and over half of these anxious respondents attributed their fear to the belief that if they did, people would be fearful of them. In April, 65 percent of those interviewed said they would keep their distance from colleagues if the latter had fevers. In July, one-sixth said they would shun colleagues who were ex-SARS patients; and one quarter said they would avoid meeting friends whose family members had been ill. Pervasive self-censorship eroded social relations in an environment already marked by lack of information and fear: 45 percent said, for example, that if they were looking for a job and if they or a relative had had SARS, they would hide the fact from potential employers. If people were willing to hide certain information from others, then they would presumably have to assume that interlocutors and strangers were likewise not disclosing everything to them, producing a climate in which everyone had to be assumed to be dangerous. That stigma could outlast the incidence of SARS and spread beyond the hospital to permeate everyday social relations is shown by the finding that 41 percent of respondents thought that ex-patients should continue to wear face masks in public places after their discharge from hospital, which would have effectively created a "marking" system by which the public could know who had been infected and siphon general fears into specific stigmatizing processes. Whereas the medically recommended period of self-quarantine before resuming normal social contact was 14 days, 33 percent of those surveyed thought it was appropriate for ex-patients to take an extended period, up to a maximum of 120 days.[29] A 44-year-old uninfected man living in Block F of the Amoy Gardens complained in a focus group: "Although it was then June, I still experienced stigmatization. I received a job order from a flat in Block Q. After I arrived at the flat, a Filipino maid followed me closely and wiped everything I touched. That was so ridiculous!"[30]

Stigma and Delegitimation

These kinds of stigma are closely related to behaviors aimed at protecting self and family from the direct threat of infection. But this is not the only form stigma takes. The indigenous Chinese model of stigma is a sociosomatic one that frames delegitimation as the central process. Traditionally, stigma extended to those who it was believed had become morally polluted by their suffering, and whose moral pollution, it was also believed, might be contagious to others, so that they and their family members also bore this kind of personal and collective loss of face. This is what Erving Goffman calls "courtesy stigma," which has the potential to affect a large number of people.[31] Thus health-care workers found that their children were isolated at schools and were themselves treated unfairly because they lived in buildings or regions in a city that were perceived to be at risk of SARS infection. Over the long term, delegitimation becomes routinized, so that patients and families are regarded as morally bankrupt and capable of bankrupting others. *Renqing*, favor, the affect central to social exchange in China can neither be given nor received.[32] Everyday moral bonds break down, and delegitimated persons are not only discriminated against and isolated but, because of their loss of face or moral worth, experience great challenges in negotiating this context, producing a cycle in which stigmatization can redouble as social exile, economic loss, and personal or familial moral degradation. Buddhist ideas of bad karma arising from previous lives and Confucian notions that loss of moral status leads to social inefficacy in one's network of connections intensify this collective sensibility, so that stigma affects not only the person but also family and social networks.

Nor is it surprising that stigma associated with SARS quickly transferred to ethnically Chinese communities in many parts of the world. This phenomenon is hardly new. There is a long tradition of Chinese being stigmatized in America as vectors of disease (i.e., venereal disease, leprosy, and other infectious diseases). For example, over a century ago, the American Medical Association sponsored a study to investigate the hypothesis that Chinese women were spreading a unique and particularly virulent strain of so-called Chinese syphilis. No evidence, of course, was found to support the claim, and yet a top publication accused the Chinese of "infusing a poison in the Anglo-Saxon bloodstream." In 1899, with the arrival of the bubonic plague in Hawaii, the local board of health quarantined Chinese residents and torched large sections of Honolulu's Chinatown. A year later, when the plague showed up in San Francisco, authorities razed Chinese neighborhoods.[33] This tradition of stigma seemed to be rekindled by the global threat of SARS. In the United States, people stayed away from Chinese restaurants. Chinese-Americans experienced distancing and avoidance.[34] President Bush's signing of an executive order allowing health authorities to forcibly quarantine people potentially infected with SARS marked, for the first time in two decades, the addition of a disease to the list of infectious illnesses that warrant detention of citizens.[35] Chinese communities in the United States felt terribly vulnerable and a target of these measures. This situation was compounded by the fact that the clinical features of SARS infection are highly nonspecific. Laboratory testing in the United States, for example, ruled out SARS-CoV infection in 100 percent of suspect cases.[36]

There were numerous cases of quarantine and overt discrimination against suspected SARS carriers around the world. In Australia, Saudi

Arabia, Italy, and Panama, to name just a few countries, travelers from Asia were subject to stringent medical checks at airports, prolonged quarantines, or barred altogether. In some areas of Russia, illegal Chinese immigrants were isolated in a work camp. "We'll give these Chinese people a piece of land," said a local bureaucrat, "and let them work there. We're going to order a special bus and ship new groups of them out there once a week."[37] Healthy disabled athletes from Hong Kong were required to be isolated from Hong Kong for ten days before going to Ireland for the Special Olympics World Summer Games.[38] The border between appropriate public health precautions based on epidemiological profiles and racial and ethnic profiling became very thin.

Between Stigma and Intervention

Obviously, the SARS epidemic was a global health crisis, which might have resulted in much greater mortality, and as such, it called for effective public health measures, some of which may have encroached on ordinary human rights. The magnitude of the potential threat justified stringent interventions, which to all appearances were effective. But we do not believe that stigmatizing sufferers contributed to the positive outcome. More likely it made control harder and less efficacious, thereby further injuring or blaming victims. There is no case to be made here for stigmatization as a rational public health intervention. Everything we know about stigma demonstrates that its effects are entirely negative.[39] The vulnerability of marginal groups to stigma is as well documented as their vulnerability to bureaucratic manipulation. It is not surprising, therefore, that in Hong Kong, SARS patients were at one point to be placed in isolation in a psychiatric hospital that accommodated legally detained psychiatric patients who could not voluntarily leave the hospital. The moral status of both groups, SARS patients and the mentally ill, was seen as similarly diminished. However, the plan was suspended, partly because of the furious discontent of residents nearby the hospital—an ironic instance of "stigma helping the stigmatized," as it were.[40]

In mainland China, economic migrants also occupy a stigmatized marginal position in large cities, despite their large numbers, and we know little about how they fared in the SARS epidemic. In rural areas, they were indeed seen as SARS vectors, and political mobilization in rural areas included the identification and isolation of migrant workers who returned home during the outbreak.[41] Again, the question is where public health security and justifiable caution give way to discrimination or abuse. The threat of infection can lead to the greater danger of people responding in excessive ways, even using violence in the name of self-protection. The interface of social experiences and bureaucratic interventions among rural populations or migrant workers is one of the most important domains for in-depth ethnographic or epidemiological research in China.

What can be learned from these experiences? For one thing, SARS creates problems for theories that explain experiences of stigma by means of a rigid "us" versus "them" binary. There is a zone of indeterminacy between those infected and those completely unaffected by SARS, which includes those indirectly connected with SARS in some way through an afflicted family member, a friend, a co-worker, or neighbors. Given the ordinariness of the symptoms, it is easy to confuse infected and uninfected persons. Nearly everyone knew an infected individual in Hong Kong, for example, but people had to hide this information because of the stigmatizing environment. Hence, because everyone was hypothetically lying and covering up, everyone was seen as potentially infected. Indeed, the psychological toll of SARS was evident from the general public. In a large-scale telephone survey, the Hong Kong Mood Disorders Center found that, in early May, one-fifth of randomly selected respondents suffered from anxiety and depression (e.g., insomnia, problems concentrating, and inability to relax). Fully, 68 percent of the respondents reported that they had persistent worries about themselves or their family members becoming infected with SARS in the previous four weeks. Fear of infecting others (57.3 percent), incurability/death (36.6 percent), and the adverse effect of SARS on job or income (17.2 percent) were the most commonly stated reasons for fearing SARS. Half of the respondents thought Hong Kong's future inauspicious.[42]

To the extent that stigma is at least partly rooted in fears, the widespread panic and somatic distress in the general population provided a fertile context in which paranoia, blaming, and scapegoating could emerge and proliferate. Mood disorders and paranoia affected not only the general public but frontline hospital staff too, thereby compromising their capacity for good clinical care. In Beijing, a study of 149 medical staff of SARS wards revealed that they were significantly more paranoid than control subjects during the outbreak. This was attributed to the discriminatory encounters that they and their families had experienced as a consequence of having worked in infected areas.[43] Chong's observations in southern Taiwan confirmed this impact on clinical staff. As a psychiatrist treating frontline hospital staff caring for SARS patients, Chong noted that anger toward the hospital administration and despair related to stigma affecting themselves and their family members surfaced in emotionally loaded debriefing sessions.[44] Stigma thus both extends outward from the hospital when ex-patients face shunning and discrimination and folds back onto the hospital by limiting the access of families to infected patients and diminishing hospital workers' capacity to provide care. In addition, it leads many people to refuse to seek help or to identify ill friends and family members.

Information Technology and the State

SARS underscored the extent to which communication technologies can propel both unreasonable fears and preventative social responses, thereby blurring the boundary between vigilance and paranoia. In

Hong Kong, before the government decided to list all the buildings with infected residents, an independent web site established on March 31 released information about the homes and workplaces of people infected in the city.[45] For the price of a one-minute phone call (about 13 cents), customers of a telecommunication company were able to call a special hotline on their mobile telephones and receive a text message listing all the buildings within a kilometer of their location that were associated with confirmed SARS cases.[46] In an attempt to build a global system of "inter-city defense" for controlling SARS more efficiently, a group of public health and bioenvironmental systems engineering experts in Taiwan proposed a sophisticated "geographic information system" whereby individuals, residential clusters, and entire communities at risk would be geospatially mapped. The computerized spatial data would then be analyzed and networked among various authorities.[47] Such a diffuse system of surveillance, while possibly effective for public health control, is also unprecedented in its potential to tightly consolidate knowledge and power and produce stigma. Confidentiality, anonymity, and other legal and human rights protections are open to compromise.

These trends partly reflect the operations of what might be called "bio-power" and the production of what Ulrich Beck terms a "world risk society." Given the role played by nongovernmental agencies such as the WHO, the Western press, Internet users, and so on, in the production of fear and the organization of effective means of controlling the epidemic, one is tempted to analyze this society in terms of "empire," in the sense in which Michael Hardt and Antonio Negri have defined it. The "paradox of power" is that the more empire envelops and invests the social field, the more global its reach becomes, the more it relinquishes its capacity to fully mediate or capture social forces. As governmental and nongovernmental agencies try to regulate the social field, they also reveal and produce different kinds of risk and new spaces for regulation.[48] However, in the Chinese context, such an analysis is somewhat misplaced. Of course, the globalization of the media and of liberal discourse played a crucial role in the epidemic, as many of the chapters in this volume note. However, as the chapters also insist, the intervention of the Chinese state was as much a "modern" biopolitical event as it was morally archaic. Ironically, the Chinese state was legitimated through its initial failure to exert control, either coercive or consensual. Nonetheless, the state's handling of the epidemic, even as it involved globalizing discourse about risk, was more centralized and focused than typically biopolitical interventions. This may say something as well about the efficacy of such interventions.

It is not hard to imagine that if SARS had not occurred in major cities, at economic and technological centers, its political management might have been different, perhaps less rapid and effective (compare, for example, the poor monitoring and treatment of infectious diseases such as malaria and tuberculosis, which kill not hundreds but millions of people in the developing world).[49] The SARS outbreak showed that governmental management of information can contribute to fear and stigma. The Chinese government's initial handling of the epidemic using the well-honed practices of secrecy and denial contributed to rumors, misunderstanding, and discrimination.[50] In Hong Kong, minority groups complained that they knew little about SARS because the government failed to broadcast information in their native languages. The government has also been widely criticized in the media for having been too slow to recognize evidence of community outbreaks of SARS and for exacerbating fear and uncertainty among the general public, a lack of biopolitical control.[51] In the absence of accurate information and honest statements about the real parameters of the epidemic, popular fear escalated as a mode of "caution" aimed at protecting families and communities. The outcome was predictable. Via a psychological defense mechanism involving labeling, marginalizing, and disavowing, stigmatization became a weapon for defending individuals and families and communities from what was unknown or erroneously known. Conditions became chaotic and fierce. People used any advantage to ward off threats. In an environment of overwhelming suspiciousness, anyone can be labeled a potential threat and face stigmatization.

China's handling of the SARS epidemic could have contributed to such paranoia. It also illustrates how public health dangers are easily eclipsed by political economic interests. The Chinese government's initial silence was in part a strategy for "keeping fear down among consumers and foreign businesses," for inhibiting discourse and knowledge about the population rather than proliferating it, because an epidemic and a travel advisory from the WHO would have been economically disastrous.[52] A detailed report about the first outbreak of SARS in Guangzhou, available in January 2003, was apparently concealed from the HKSAR.[53] The situation changed after a few visits to heavily infected cities in China by a team of investigators deployed by the WHO. Once organized policies and programs were substituted for secrecy and denial, popular energy shifted dramatically under the timely mobilization efforts of the propaganda machine. Doctors and nurses, the former sources of fear and pollution, became heroic fighters toiling at the front, even as they still faced ongoing stigma in their local worlds. "It's humiliating," said one nurse, "We are doing a job that other people do not want to do and yet we are treated like this."[54]

Destigmatization and the Problems of Social Control

Knowledge of the course of SARS infection and its treatment lessened (though it did not by any means remove) the fear of discharged patients and their families. But attention to the emotional, moral, and social effects of SARS has been limited, and the propaganda apparatus did not focus on the aftermath of SARS as a means of providing accurate and full information in the effort to destigmatize SARS patients. Anna Wu, the former chair of the Equal Opportunities Commission (EOC) of Hong Kong, emphasized that there was not enough information stating that recovered SARS patients need not be feared.[55] Likewise, the *South China Morning Post* editorialized in late July: "The government must step up its efforts to educate the public about the myths, as well as the dangers, of SARS. Most of the information available . . . deals with preventing the spread of the disease. . . . But there is little information to reassure the recovered SARS patient who wants friends and workmates to know that he or she does not pose a risk."[56]

Stigma opens a window on Chinese social and cultural practices. For all the enormous change that Chinese people have undergone, the nexus of moral-emotional processes that have traditionally made loss of face so central to the Chinese experience seems to be as intact as ever. This moral-emotional core of Chinese culture fuels stigmatization and creates the largest barrier to destigmatization. While public information campaigns can sometimes improve public attitudes, stigma can become deeply entrenched through cultural beliefs and moral convictions. It can be intensified through less apparent and more pernicious structural forms of discrimination, where social policies and bureaucratic procedures systematically work against stigmatized persons. And yet experiences of stigma can also lead to the creation of new social sympathies and affiliations. Overseas Chinese formed associations to work against the stigmatization of Chinese and Chinese businesses due to SARS.[57] Many SARS sufferers have received emotional and financial support from family members. Many sufferers have come to sympathize with strangers also facing stigmatization. "I want justice," said an uninfected woman in Hong Kong who was rejected for residency elsewhere simply because she had previously lived in an affected area. "I am a completely healthy person, but I still faced such unfair treatment. I can just imagine the social discrimination against those who actually came down with SARS, their families, and the frontline medical workers."[58]

The global public health manpower expended on finding, isolating, and quarantining cases of SARS was almost unprecedented in the history of infectious diseases. If all of this is to be seen cynically by those fearful of the ever-tentacular reaches of social control and bio-power, SARS and its management also raised new ethical and moral questions regarding the often necessary uses of social control. Where practices like quarantine and surveillance are absolutely necessary, one must also inquire into the negative and positive effects that public health interventions produce over time, how effects become durable social experiences for people and either bolster or undermine the capacity of governmental and nongovernmental agencies to operate in the world.

The central issues for public health policy have been to provide access to health services that can deliver effective treatment and to identify and isolate carriers of SARS to combat transmission of the infection. Isolation and quarantine were absolutely essential aspects of the public health control of SARS. Yet we can also learn from the ways in which such practices created new injuries and dilemmas for sufferers. Stigma contributes to the factors, such as fear and isolation, that allow quarantine to operate properly. But there is a downside to quarantine, one that can undermine public health. For example, quarantine limits early case identification by causing people to keep quiet about symptoms. Quarantine may compound suffering where it produces unnecessary kinds of avoidance, discrimination, and isolation, and where familial and social networks are broken. In such cases, not only do sufferers confront stigma that lessens their life chances and intensifies their pain, but the traditional channels of emotional care and financial support are also eroded.

Stigmatizing SARS is closely associated with the fear of becoming infected and therefore being put at risk of death. Yet this fear, like those of other stigmatized illnesses, is disproportionate to the medically assessed risk of SARS. Global telecommunications, including the mass media, have played a formative role in fueling this fear. In this context, what is now being called "lay epidemiology" can dominate, where speculations animated by paranoia quickly pass as science and animate social policies that reproduce rather than remedy stigmatized conditions. For example, in May 2003, a German newspaper, receiving a number of inquiries from doctors concerned about doing business in Asia, predicted that in two years all of Hong Kong would be infected with SARS, ignoring interventions that decrease the contact rate and transmission probability, and, as noted, animating stigmatizing social reactions.[59]

These two faces of quarantine are not easily disentangled and are often mutually constitutive. In fact, the extant theories on stigma support this state of entanglement. T. F. Heatherton et al. have, for example, proposed a multidimensional framework to situate stigma from the perspectives of the stigmatizer (perceiver), the stigmatized (perceived), and the context of stigmatization. According to this conceptual frame, the views and experiences of the perceivers and the perceived can be at variance with each other and must be simultaneously considered in understanding and preventing stigma in a particular setting.[60] Thus, from the perspectives of the state, health organizations, employers, and the general public, quarantine is justifiable. A focus group conducted by Sing Lee et al. in Hong Kong revealed that members of the general public generally rationalized the stigmatizing treatment of Amoy Gardens residents or ex-SARS subjects as "cautiousness." A 27-year-old dietitian said, "I remembered that I had rejected dining with a friend who recovered from SARS, but I do not think that avoiding someone who may infect others constitutes discrimination; only shunning those who look ugly or have mental illness is." Fear of economic setbacks rationalized people's costly precautionary measures. A 32-year-old woman pointed out: "Overseas clients refused to come to Hong Kong and so we had to spend U.S.$5.6 a minute to conduct video-conferencing meetings." A middle-aged woman said: "I arranged for every worker to have daily temperature checks and to have chest X-rays in order to make sure that the factory could operate as usual. I could not afford to be careless, because the detection of one single case of suspected SARS would mean the entire factory would have to be closed." Finally, a 46-year-old owner of several restaurants that suffered financial losses during the SARS outbreak said: "It is unfair to call the stringent health measures we took discrimination. They are only to protect oneself. Ex-SARS patients themselves have the responsibility to be cautious about infecting others."[61]

But quarantine and other preventative measures are inherently stigmatizing. Indeed, one might say that if there ever were an appropriate use of stigma in public health policy, SARS would be it. But this conventional argument—that stigma finds its positive utilitarian dimension in quarantine—is neither convincing nor acceptable. There is no question that quarantine is a necessary and useful preventative strategy for public health, but its proponents must find alternative ways of legitimating its implementation and dealing with its less than desirable and potentially dangerous social consequences. This may be the most important lesson related to SARS—that the problem of social stigma is intimately tied to health system responses. How does one conduct quarantine and, at the same time, limit as much as possible these negative social and psychological consequences? How does one conduct quarantine without, at the same time, undermining that intervention by producing popular fears, inducing cultures of secrecy, and limiting case identification?

Health care, especially prevention and public health, has been low on the list of policy priorities among most Asian governments, which, in an attempt to focus on economic growth, spend a much lower portion of their GDP on health care than their Western counterparts. Unsurprisingly, the SARS crisis has uncovered multiple inadequacies and failings of their health-care systems. In response to the media's vigorous attempts to indict such inefficiency, government and professional spokesmen could have defensively communicated an inflated risk of SARS to the public at large. In frequent news briefing sessions, they highlighted mortality figures, individuals, buildings, and local communities that required quarantine, the importance of frequent hand-washing and other precautionary procedures. The information they thus conveyed (continued spread, mortality despite public health measures) and the feeling of bleakness that accompanied their replies to reporters, contributed to an overwhelmingly frightening perception of the impact of SARS. That, of course, bred stigma.

In the "2003 Asia Pacific Inter-city SARS Forum" held in Taipei after the SARS crisis was over, Chi-pon Wen, a professor at the National Health Research Institute, Taiwan, addressed the topic of "risk communication." In his view, the enormous gap between the "perceived" risk and "assessed" risk of SARS resulted in unnecessarily "expensive lessons" for Taiwan. He emphasized that the media focus throughout the crisis was unbalanced, centered on myths about SARS, panic, and hasty responses. He suggested more effective ways of providing risk communication to the public that might minimize rumor and panic during future outbreaks. Making valid risk comparisons (e.g., motorcycle accidents and suicide claimed 4,000 and 2,200 lives a year in Taiwan, but SARS only 71) and managing misperceptions about risk, Wen proposed, would go a long way toward producing more efficient and equitable responses.

In the winter of 2004–5, there was a reemergence of SARS in southern China, with three case identifications. It is not clear how and why SARS came back, although wild and domesticated animals were seen as a likely source. China continued to take substantial preventative measures, such as the killing of civet cats raised and sold commercially. Whether or not these preventative measures are helping to put off a larger reappearance of SARS is unclear, although it is clear that SARS will be around for a while, probably existing at low levels but potentially flashing up again. In the winter, Chinese doctors began administering a SARS vaccine to volunteers. If effective, this would be a significant step toward reducing the threat of another outbreak. Yet during the winter of 2004–5, there was also an avian flu epidemic in Southeast Asia. These two epidemics cannot be seen as isolated phenomena. The successes with regard to the one are counterbalanced by the threats posed by the other, such that in today's international milieu, it appears as if one infectious disease can be easily supplanted by another. Taken together, all emerging infectious diseases must be seen in the context of global interconnection, national and international responses, as well as in relation to other infectious diseases, such as the Ebola virus, and the production of stigmatizing conditions that are not specific to particular diseases but come to impact communities and regions.

Implications for Health and Social Policy

Framing SARS in terms of social stigma and social suffering suggests that to improve the quality of life and reduce suffering, as well as to produce positive and efficient public health outcomes, it is essential that health and social policy address stigma and the social and cultural processes through which discrimination becomes routine. One patients' rights group in Hong Kong has demanded that the Hospital Authority provide more emotional support for sufferers. The Hospital Authority did not allow family members to visit SARS patients during the epidemic, taking a "huge psychological toll" among patients, including cases of clinical depression. "SARS patients are isolated from their families and their community," said Jim Pang Hung-Cheon, a spokesperson for the patients' rights group. "Doctors and nurses can only offer them medical treatment but not emotional support. For some people, their family members were admitted to hospitals and then died. They could not see each other during this period. This was a terrible experience."[62] Systematic efforts at destigmatization are crucial at this stage. Unfortunately, not much is known about how to conduct public health practices in a way that does not inevitably result in stigma. This is particularly true in China, where normative social and cultural processes, as well as core moral and emotional convictions, are especially conducive to stigma. These problems will demand long-term ethnographic and public health research.

From the perspective of research, the evolving biosocial course of

SARS offers a special window on the topic of stigma.[63] Uncertain routes of transmission, unknown effects on the nonclinical population, controversial medical methods of treatment, and likelihood of reemergence remain characteristics of SARS. It also seems increasingly likely that laboratory tests for SARS-CoV infection with good sensitivity and specificity will soon be available. This will reduce the number of individuals falsely suspected of having contracted SARS but may also detect a large number of seropositive (and therefore potentially stigmatizable) individuals in the community among whom the course of the illness remains unclear. James Chin has reviewed threatening nonpandemic viral infections over the past century. Believing that the SARS outbreak died out without quarantine procedures in Guangdong (where the first known SARS outbreak occurred but was apparently concealed), he concludes that although the reemergenceof SARS infections is unlikely, it cannot be ruled out.[64] Others expect reemergence as well, but in a limited form. Whatever the future course of SARS, unnecessary fears could be eased if more accurate information were available. Already, by July, when the SARS outbreak was over, negative attitudes and behaviors toward SARS had decreased in Hong Kong. But stigma has persisted in a subgroup of individuals who appear to hold intractable discriminatory attitudes.[65]

The social dimension of suffering constitutes much of what is meant by prognosis. SARS sufferers and their families need programs that can respond to the psychological aspects of their suffering and inhibit the further development of mental illnesses and social strife. In communities, workplaces, and schools, destigmatization can only occur through effective policies and proactive programs aimed at addressing the everyday fears and moral convictions that sustain stigma. Because potentially discriminatory practices are couched in the language of public health and corporate risk management, destigmatizing SARS may be a particularly trying project. Essential aspects of this will include providing accurate and accessible information to the public; speaking truth to rumor and falsehood; protecting the legal rights and privacy of individuals and families; health education programs; advocacy for patients' rights; training of primary care practitioners; community action projects; networking with the media to communicate risk in idioms that are grounded but not reactionary; guidelines for human resources managers to build strategies that safeguard both legitimate corporate interests and employee rights; and programs that help former patients reenter society. Only by combining social and health policies, social and health services, social experience and hard numbers can we adequately address the many dimensions of suffering that confront SARS patients and their families, and evade the pernicious cycles of stigma that compound affliction, inhibit recovery, create workplace difficulties, and undermine public health programs and policies.

CHAPTER TEN

SARS and the Consequences for Globalization

JAMES L. WATSON

The essays in this book demonstrate that the 2002–2003 SARS outbreak can be read in a variety of ways. Economists and political scientists see it as a temporary setback in China's drive to join the global economy. As a social anthropologist who focuses on the cultural aspects of globalization, I take a different view.

The events of the winter of 2003 might best be seen as a warning shot, a wake-up call for security officials, economic planners, and policymakers—everywhere, not just in China. SARS, combined with the events following 9/11, forces us to reexamine many of the optimistic, utopian visions of globalization that emerged during the 1990s. This chapter looks at infectious diseases as a *potential* inhibiting factor in the future of globalization and international migration.

Readers will no doubt recall the euphoria of the dot.com era, when the U.S. stock market was booming and investors were assured by pundits that the digital revolution was creating a "New Economy." Twentieth-century business cycles and market crashes were consigned to the rubbish bin of history. The optimism, the naïveté, of that era encouraged a whole generation of theorists to write about the disappearance of the state, the irrelevance of borders, and the transformative power of the Internet.

During the 1990s, the pages of *Foreign Affairs*, the world's leading policy studies journal, were filled with articles on globalization, most of which challenged the received wisdom of earlier generations. Publishers could not find enough manuscripts to satisfy an international readership that would buy anything with the word "global" in its title. By mid 2004, however, the market for such products had collapsed as affluent readers began to face the boomerang effects of globalization—including the "offshore outsourcing" of high-tech, digital-savvy jobs.[1] In its March 2004 issue, *Harper's Magazine* announced "The Death of Globalization"—the tide was turning.[2]

Is globalization in fact dead? And, if so, was SARS one of the angels of death? To paraphrase Mark Twain, it would be foolhardy to celebrate the demise of globalization at the first signs of illness.[3] Views of globalism depend upon one's political perspective: Should we focus on the victims or the victors of global capitalism? Are yesterday's losers tomorrow's winners, as recent critics of the offshoring of U.S. jobs to China and India maintain?[4]

In hindsight, the utopian writings of the late 1990s seem curiously outmoded, even though they were produced only a few short years ago. One of the best examples is Richard Rosencrance's 1999 book *The Rise of the Virtual State: Wealth and Power in the Coming Century*. The title captures the revolutionary optimism of the era: according to Rosencrance, information flows will increase rapidly in the twenty-first century as the need for military intervention dissipates (or it evolves into police actions). Control over knowledge and technology will be more important than domination of land and territory. To be fair, Rosencrance argues that these are long-term projections that follow the inevitable logic of globalization and digitization.[5]

Perhaps the most radical of the dot.com theorists is Kevin Kelly, former executive editor of *Wired* magazine and guru to the 1990s digerati. In his influential book *Out of Control: The New Biology of Machines, Social Systems, and the Economic World,* Kelly spoke for the rapidly expanding community of web enthusiasts.[6] He predicted that the Internet would gradually erode the power of governments to control citizens; in Kelly's view, digital technology made it possible for transstate coalitions to thrive in cyberspace.

In the 1990s, *Wired* published a steady stream of articles that envisioned a world characterized by continuous, uninhibited access to information. This, in turn, would render obsolete the many twentieth-century ideologies founded on notions of ethnicity, religion, and class. *Wired* subscribers who were veterans of the 1960s student movements could not help but notice the parallels to earlier, Marxian dreams of a classless, stateless world. In its heyday, *Wired* was the hackers' equivalent of *The Communist Manifesto*; even the language of Engels and Marx's 1848 broadside finds parallels in the "netizen" screeds published in the 1990s.[7]

Not surprisingly, many anthropologists were affected by the digital revolution and its visions of an open, free-flowing global system. One of the most interesting anthropological discourses on globalization is Arjun Appadurai's *Modernity at Large: Cultural Dimensions of Globalization*, published at the height of the dot.com boom.[8] Appadurai focuses on highly educated English-speaking professionals who were born in South Asia and emigrated to Europe or the United States, where they have spent their adult years. Migratory elites create what Appadurai refers to as "diasporic public spheres" that cut across state borders and link people in real-time communication networks (cell phones, email, rapid air travel). Contemporary diasporas of this type are not just transnational, they are "postnational," to use Appadurai's apt phrase—meaning that the people who operate in these spheres are oblivious to national borders and maintain multiple home bases.[9]

Another anthropological study that tracked diasporic elites is *Flexible Citizenship: The Cultural Logics of Transnationality*, by Aihwa Ong.[10] Ong's subjects are Chinese entrepreneurs, scientists, business executives, and movers and shakers in the world of global finance. The book's title reflects the lifestyle of these elites, captured at a critical moment during the mid-1990s economic boom. This was a period when it was relatively easy for people to hold multiple citizenships and to fly across the Pacific several times each year without worrying about immigration controls on either side.

The disaporics described by Appadurai and Ong are living examples of postmodernism—defined (for the purposes of this essay) as a lifestyle conditioned by the collapse of time and space.[11] Contemporary travelers experience this implosion in a very vivid, direct, and personal manner. In the late 1960s, for instance, a telephone call from Hong Kong to London cost approximately U.S.$10 per minute, assuming one could find a line that handled international "trunk" calls. Today, the same call can be made for pennies, and there is no shortage of competitive cell phone options. Meanwhile, air travel has become a routine experience for millions of middle- and working-class migrants. The price of a transoceanic ticket has declined severalfold since the 1960s (allowing for inflation), while incomes have increased sharply. Appadurai's and Ong's diasporics could not help but feel that state borders had become "porous," in striking contrast to the perceived experience of their parents' generation of migrants.[12]

Will post-9/11 political developments make these late-twentieth-century lifestyles seem hopelessly out of step with twenty-first century political realities? Evidence now points to an era of *hard-boundaried* states, reinforced by increasing border surveillance and visa barriers that restrict the free flow of people. Flexible or multiple citizenships may be a thing of the past. This seems especially true in the uncertain aftermath of the Iraq War and the rise of terrorism in Europe and the Middle East. Who, at this point, would dare predict what the emerging global system will look like?

This brings us to SARS.

The reemergence of open, porous borders seems even more unlikely given the developments of winter 2003. It can be argued that the SARS outbreak—and, by implication, the prospect of similar epidemics in the future—presents a more serious challenge to the openness of the global system than the September 2001 terrorism attacks on New York and Washington. Americans watched live CNN images of U.S. border controls hardening after 9/11; even remote crossings on the Canadian border seized up for a time as automobiles and trucks were rigorously inspected. At U.S. airports, the immigration queues for noncitizens slowed to a "snail's pace" (to quote one British colleague). Visas for young men from Muslim-majority countries were effectively frozen, and hundreds of Chinese students arrived late for graduate school during the fall semester of 2002.

As painful as were the tragic events of September 11, 2001, the subsequent border-disrupting effects were selective, temporary, and partial. The response to international terrorism produced nothing like the complete and utterly indiscriminate shutdown associated with SARS. There was no selective profiling of suspected SARS carriers. The winter 2003 embargo on travel to and from epidemic hot spots lasted for weeks in some cases.

The full chronology of the SARS episode is covered in the Introduction to this book. The epidemic appears to have "gone global" on or around February 28, 2003, when an outbreak of flulike symptoms was reported in Hanoi. Severe acute respiratory syndrome, or SARS, as it later became known, was linked to a business traveler who arrived in Vietnam from Guangdong province in southern China.[13]

The World Health Organization (WHO) headquarters in Geneva issued a global health alert on March 12 in response to the spread of SARS to Hong Kong and Toronto (see chapter 2). Prior to this notification, the most recent WHO global alert was announced in 1994, following an outbreak of plague in India.[14]

A few examples taken from media reports of the time will illustrate the threat that SARS presented to the global system:

1. On March 18, 2003, a doctor who had treated SARS patients in Singapore flew to New York. After his brief visit, he boarded a return flight to Singapore from JFK Airport; the Boeing 747 had 400 people aboard, representing fifteen countries. All 400 were quarantined in Frankfurt, an intermediate stop. There was no evidence of SARS among them.[15]

2. Passengers aboard Air China's March 15, 2003, Flight 112 from Hong Kong to Beijing were not so fortunate. A 72-year-old man with SARS was on that flight and infected at least 21 people—who spread the disease north to Inner Mongolia and south to Thailand.[16]

3. The majority of Taiwan's SARS cases can be traced to a single patient who was misdiagnosed at an early stage in the epidemic.[17]

4. At the height of the SARS scare, the occupancy rate of Hong Kong's major hotels fell to 5 percent, and it was rumored that, on some nights in April 2003, two of the territory's grandest hotels did not have a single guest.[18]

5. During the outbreak in Singapore, an internationally known bank segregated employees into three groups. The first group worked in the central office in Singapore's central banking district, the second moved to a remote site some miles away, and the third worked from home. Senior managers made it a practice *not* to meet together in the same room at the same time. Most significantly, visits to clients abroad ceased entirely, given that each trip required a 10-day quarantine at the entry port. Elaborate crisis preparations the bank had installed in the aftermath of 9/11 did not work as well as expected—disease had trumped terrorism. The executive director of the American Chamber of Commerce in Singapore put it this way: SARS is "like a neutron bomb. It affects people, not equipment."[19]

What can we conclude from these events? First, as the Singapore case illustrates, SARS threatened to kill a very large number of people; it did not affect technology or communications. The epidemic disrupted the flow of people across borders—and it was precisely the diasporic elites studied by Appadurai and Ong who were hit hardest.

SARS also tells us something important about the future of global security. Jeanne Guillemin, a specialist on bioterrorism, notes that biological warfare "by humans against humans has been rare and historically inconsequential."[20] Rather, it is "natural" biological events, brought about by the vagaries of human-animal-microbial interactions that represent the true threat to international mobility. In the end, as noted by several authors in this volume, SARS was a minor incident compared to more lethal biological events, such as the "Spanish Flu" of 1918. Historical evidence now suggests that upwards of 100 million people died during that epidemic; 20 million may have died in India alone.[21]

The cauldron for the production of global flu epidemics is the same microregion where SARS first appeared—the Pearl River Delta of Guangdong province, adjoining Hong Kong. This is an ecozone where pigs, ducks, chickens, and miscellaneous other livestock (including the now notorious civet cat) live cheek-by-jowl with farmers—in one of the planet's most densely populated regions.[22] It is here also that avian flu is currently brewing (as these words are being written in early 2005). Avian flu has already made the species jump from chickens to humans in Vietnam, south China, and the Netherlands.[23] Recent WHO and CDC warnings about the possible consequences of this jump sound ominously like what the SARS outbreak might have become under different circumstances. Homo sapiens was lucky in 2003.

Globalization is a process that is replete with ironies. One of those ironies hides behind the SARS crisis: a premodern agricultural system—based on pigs, ducks, chickens, and centuries-old technology—could well turn out to be the greatest threat to the postmodern global system.

Reference Matter

Notes

Kleinman and Watson: Introduction

1. Hans Troedsson and Anton Rychener, "When Influenza Takes Flight," *New York Times*, Feb. 5, 2005, A31.

2. Alvin So and Ngai Pun, "Globalization and Anti-Globalization of SARS in Chinese Societies," *Asian Perspective* 28, no. 1 (2004): 5–17.

3. "Singapore Man Confirmed with SARS," CNN.Com, Sept. 9, 2003.

4. See, e.g., Li Zhang, *Strangers in the City: Reconfigurations of Space, Power, and Social Networks Within China's Floating Population* (Stanford: Stanford University Press, 2001).

5. Jun Jing and Joan Kaufman, "China and AIDS: The Time to Act Is Now," *Science* 296, no. 5577 (June 28, 2002): 2339–40.

6. Abigail Kuger, "What Can We Learn from AIDS?" *New York Times*, Nov. 11, 2003, D11; Arthur Kleinman, Veena Das, and Margaret Lock, eds., *Social Suffering* (Berkeley: University of California Press, 1997).

7. The work of Michel Foucault is certainly relevant to this discussion: see his *History of Sexuality, Vol. 1: An Introduction*, trans. Robert Hurley (New York: Vintage Books, 1978), and *Madness and Civilization: A History of Insanity in the Age of Reason* (reprint, London: Routledge, 2001). And see also Adriana Petryna *Life Exposed: Biological Citizens after Chernobyl* (Princeton, N.J.: Princeton University Press, 2002), and Paul Rabinow, *Making PCR: A Story of Biotechnology* (Chicago: University of Chicago Press, 1996).

8. James Maguire, "SARS in China: CDC Official Maguire Describes the Story of What Happened," *Harvard Public Health Now*, Nov. 14, 2003 (www/hsph.harvard.edu/now/nov14/index.html).

9. Joseph Fewsmith, "Chinese Politics under Hu Jintao: Riding the Tiger of

Politics and Public Health," *Problems of Post-Communism* 50, no. 5 (2003): 14–21; see also Jonathan Mirsky, "How the Chinese Spread SARS," *New York Review of Books*, May 29, 2003, 42.

10. Maguire, "SARS in China."

11. Ibid.

12. Matt Pottinger, "Scientists Expect Bird Flu to Pose Long-Term Fight," *Wall Street Journal.com*, Feb. 7, 2005.

13. Kaylin 2003: 27.

14. Ibid.

15. There were twenty-seven probable cases in the United States, "only a handful of which were confirmed," according to the CDC's James Maguire ("SARS in China").

16. Alvin Powell, "Unknown Feeds Public Fear of SARS," *Harvard Gazette*, Apr. 10, 2003 (on-line archives).

17. Lawrence Atman, "What Is the Next Plague?" *New York Times*, Nov. 11, 2003, D8.

18. "University Lifts Travel Moratorium for Vietnam and Toronto," *Harvard Gazette*, May 1, 2003 (on-line archives).

19. Arthur Kleinman, "The Background and Development of Public Health in China: An Exploratory Essay," in *Public Health in the People's Republic of China*, ed. Myron E. Wegman, Tsung-yi Lim, and Elizabeth F. Purcell (New York: Josiah Macy, Jr. Foundation, 1973), 5–23.

20. Ibid., 10–11.

21. AnElissa Lucas, *Chinese Medical Modernization: Comparative Policy Continuities, 1930s–1980s* (New York: Praeger, 1982), 18.

22. D. R. Phillips, *The Epidemiological Transition in Hong Kong*, Center for Asian Studies Monograph No. 751 (Hong Kong: University of Hong Kong, 1988), 42.

23. Ibid., 43.

24. Kleinman, "Background and Development of Public Health in China."

25. Lucas, *Chinese Medical Modernization*, 58–64.

26. Karen Minden, *Bamboo Stone: The Evolution of Chinese Medical Elite* (Toronto: University of Toronto Press, 1994), 42.

27. C. C. Chen, *Medicine in Rural China: A Personal Account* (Berkeley: University of California Press, 1989), 122–23.

28. S. M. Hillier, "Preventative Health Work in the People's Republic of

China, 1949–1982," in *Health Care and Traditional Medicine in China, 1800–1982,* ed. S. M. Hillier and J. A. Jewell (London: Routledge, 1983), 153.

29. Kurt Deuschle, "Common Disease Patterns," in *Rural Health in the People's Republic of China: Report of a Visit by the Rural Health Systems Delegation, June 1978,* NIH Publication 81–2124 (Washington, D.C.: Department of Health and Human Services, National Institutes of Health, 1980), 5.

30. William Foege, "Surveillance and Antiepidemic Work," in *Rural Health in the People's Republic of China: Report of a Visit by the Rural Health Systems Delegation, June 1978,* NIH Publication 81–2124 (Washington, D.C.: Department of Health and Human Services, National Institutes of Health, 1980), 97.

31. Cf. Kun-Yen Huang, "Infectious and Parasitic Diseases," in *Medicine and Public Health in the People's Republic of China,* ed. Joseph R. Quinn (Washington, D.C.: Department of Health and Human Services, 1972), 239–57.

32. Foege, "Surveillance and Antiepidemic Work," 98.

33. Ibid., 97.

34. Hillier, "Preventative Health Work in the People's Republic of China, 1949–1982," 155.

35. Ibid., 156.

36. Ibid., 192.

37. Ibid., 158.

38. Ibid., 157.

39. Robert M. Worth, "New China's Accomplishments in the Control of Diseases," in *Public Health in the People's Republic of China,* ed. Myron E. Wegman, Tsung-yi Lin, and Elizabeth F. Purcell (New York: Josiah Macy, Jr. Foundation, 1973), 176–77.

40. Lucas, *Chinese Medical Modernization,* 107.

41. Susan B. Rifkin, "Health Care for Rural Areas," in *Medicine and Public Health in the People's Republic of China,* ed. Joseph R. Quinn (Washington, D.C.: Department of Health and Human Services, 1972), 137.

42. Lucas, *Chinese Medical Modernization,* 108; Minden, *Bamboo Stone.*

43. Francis L. K. Hsu, "A Cholera Epidemic in a Chinese Town," in *Health, Culture and Community: Case Studies of Public Reactions to Health Programs,* ed. Benjamin D. Paul (New York: Russell Sage Foundation, 1955), 136.

44. Ibid., 144.

45. Ibid., 145.

46. Ibid., 136.

47. During ordinary times, funeral processions were designed to draw maximum attention to the mourners; see James L. Watson, "The Structure of Chinese Funerary Rites," in *Death Ritual in Late Imperial and Modern China*, ed. James L. Watson and Evelyn S. Rawski (Berkeley: University of California Press, 1988).

48. Hsu, "Cholera Epidemic," 144.

49. Joseph Bosco, "Magic Masks and Digital Thermometers: Science and Magic in the SARS Crisis in Hong Kong" (Working Paper, Department of Anthropology, Chinese University of Hong Kong, 2004).

50. Yuqun Liao, "Thoughts about 'Local Disease' in China," in *Medicine and the History of the Body*, ed. Yasuo Otsuka, Shizu Sakai, and Shigehisa Kuriyama (Tokyo: Ishiyaku EuroAmerica, 1999), 90.

51. Randolph Schmid, "U.S. Prepares to Test Vaccine for Bird Flu," *Boston Globe*, Feb. 25, 2005, A10; "Vietnam Confirms Another Fatality from Bird Flu," *Wall Street Journal.com*, Feb. 28, 2005; David P. Hamilton and Gautam Naik, "Avian Flu Poses Challenge to Global Vaccine Industry," *Wall Street Journal.com*, Feb. 28, 2005.

1. Murray: The Epidemiology of SARS

1. Drosten C, Gunther S, Preiser W, van der Werf S, Brodt HR, Becker S, Rabenau H, Panning M, Kolesnikova L, Fouchier RA, Berger A, Burguiere AM, Cinatl J, Eickmann M, Escriou N, Grywna K, Kramme S, Manuguerra JC, Muller S, Rickerts V, Sturmer M, Vieth S, Klenk HD, Osterhaus AD, Schmitz H, Doerr HW. Identification of a novel coronavirus in patients with severe acute respiratory syndrome. *N Engl J Med*, 2003; 348: 1967–76.

2. Poutanen SM, Low DE, Henry B, Finkelstein S, Rose D, Green K, Tellier R, Draker R, Adachi D, Ayers M, Chan AK, Skowronski DM, Salit I, Simor AE, SlutskyAS, Doyle PW, Krajden M, Petric M, Brunham RC, McGeer AJ; National Microbiology Laboratory, Canada; Canadian Severe Acute Respiratory Syndrome Study Team. Identification of severe acute respiratory syndrome in Canada. *N Engl J Med*, 2003; 348: 1995–2005.

3. Marra MA, Jones SJ, Astell CR, Holt RA, Brooks-Wilson A, Butterfield YS, Khattra J, Asano JK, Barber SA, Chan SY, Cloutier A, Coughlin SM, Freeman D, Girn N, Griffith OL, Leach SR, Mayo M, McDonald H, Montgomery SB, Pandoh PK, Petrescu AS, Robertson AG, Schein JE, Siddiqui A, Smailus DE, Stott JM, Yang GS, Plummer F, Andonov A, Artsob H, Bastien N, Bernard K, Booth TF, Bowness D, Czub M, Drebot M, Fernando L, Flick R, Garbutt M, Gray M,

Grolla A, Jones S, Feldmann H, Meyers A, Kabani A, Li Y, Normand S, Stroher U, Tipples GA, Tyler S, Vogrig R, Ward D, Watson B, Brunham RC, Krajden M, Petric M, Skowronski DM, Upton C, Roper RL. The Genome sequence of the SARS-associated coronavirus. *Science*, 2003; 300(5624): 1399–1404.

4. Rota PA, Oberste MS, Monroe SS, Nix WA, Campagnoli R, Icenogle JP, Penaranda S, Bankamp B, Maher K, Chen MH, Tong S, Tamin A, Lowe L, Frace M, DeRisi JL, Chen Q, Wang D, Erdman DD, Peret TC, Burns C, Ksiazek TG, Rollin PE, Sanchez A, Liffick S, Holloway B, Limor J, McCaustland K, Olsen-Rasmussen M, Fouchier R, Gunther S, Osterhaus AD, Drosten C, Pallansch MA, Anderson LJ, Bellini WJ. Characterization of a novel coronavirus associated with severe acute respiratory syndrome. *Science*, 2003; 300(5624): 1394–99.

5. Wickramasinghe C, Wainwright M, Narlikar J. SARS—a clue to its origins? *Lancet*, 2003; 361(9371): 1832.

6. "Update: Multistate Outbreak of Monkeypox—Illinois, Indiana, Kansas, Missouri, Ohio, and Wisconsin, 2003," *Morbidity and Mortality Weekly Report*, 52, no. 27 (July 11, 2003): 642–46, http://www.cdc.gov/mmwr/PDF/wk/mm5227.pdf (accessed Apr. 6, 2005).

7. Seto WH, Tsang D, Yung RW, Ching TY, Ng TK, Ho M, Ho LM, Peiris JS; Advisors of Expert SARS group of Hospital Authority. Effectiveness of precautions against droplets and contact in prevention of nosocomial transmission of severe acute respiratory syndrome (SARS). *Lancet*, 2003; 361(9368): 1519–20.

8. Dwosh HA, Hong HH, Austgarden D, Herman S, Schabas R. Identification and containment of an outbreak of SARS in a community hospital. *CMAJ*, 2003; 168: 1415–20.

9. Ng SK. Possible role of an animal vector in the SARS outbreak at Amoy Gardens. *Lancet*, 2003; 362(9383): 570–72.

10. Lipsitch M, Cohen T, Cooper B, Robins JM, Ma S, James L, Gopalakrishna G, Chew SK, Tan CC, Samore MH, Fisman D, Murray M. Transmission dynamics and control of severe acute respiratory syndrome. *Science*, 2003; 300(5627): 1966–70.

11. Riley S, Fraser C, Donnelly CA, Ghani AC, Abu-Raddad LJ, Hedley AJ, Leung GM, Ho LM, Lam TH, Thach TQ, Chau P, Chan KP, Lo SV, Leung PY, Tsang T, Ho W, Lee KH, Lau EM, Ferguson NM, Anderson RM. Transmission dynamics of the etiological agent of SARS in Hong Kong: impact of public health interventions. *Science*, 2003; 300: 1961–66.

12. "Sars and Emerging Zoonoses," WHO/CDS/GAR, Nov. 2003.

13. Low DE. Why SARS will not return: a polemic. *CMAJ*, 2004; 170: 68–69.

2. Schnur: The Role of the WHO

1. International Health Regulations, WHO Geneva, 1969. In May 2005 the World Health Assembly passed resolution WHA58.3 adopting revised international health regulations. The revised regulations will formally come into force two years from the date on which the Assembly approved them (http://www.who.int/gb/ebwha/pdf_files/WHA58/WHA58_3-en.pdf [accessed July 25, 2005].

2. WHO WPRO mission report on a visit to southern China, Jan. 16–23, 1998, Dr. Koichi Morita, WHO Manila.

3. Law of the People's Republic of China on the Prevention and Control of Contagious Disease, Sixth Meeting of the Standing Committee of the Seventh National People's Congress, Feb. 21, 1989; G. Zeng, J. Zhang, K. Rou, et al., "Infectious Disease Surveillance in China," *Biomedical and Environmental Sciences* (Beijing) 11 (1998): 31–37.

4. WHO China email sent to MOH and WHO WPRO, Feb. 10, 2003.

5. Acute respiratory syndrome in Hong Kong Special Administrative Region of China/ Vietnam, Mar. 12, 2003 (www.who.int/csr/don/2003_03_12/en [accessed Apr. 25, 2005]).

6. Severe Acute Respiratory Syndrome (SARS)—multi-country outbreak, Mar. 15 2003 (www.who.int/csr/don/2003_03_15/en [accessed Apr. 25, 2005]).

7. Robert F. Breiman, Meirion Evans, Wolfgang Preiser, et al., "Role of China in the Quest to Define and Control Severe Acute Respiratory Syndrome," *Journal of Emerging Infectious Diseases* 9, no. 9 (September 2003): 1037–41; Ruiheng Xu, JianFeng He, Meirion R. Evans, et al., "Epidemiologic Clues to SARS Origin in China," *Emerging Infectious Diseases 10*, no. 6 (June 2004):1030–37.

8. WHO Mission report on a visit to Guangdong province to review the SARS situation, Apr. 3–8, 2003 (unpublished report, WHO China office).

9. WHO Mission report on a visit to Beijing municipality to review the SARS situation, Apr. 11–15, 2003 (unpublished report, WHO China office).

10. World Health Assembly Resolution on Severe Acute Respiratory Syndrome (SARS), WHA56.29, May 28, 2003 (http://www.who.int/gb/ebwha/pdf_files/WHA56/ea56r29.pdf [accessed Apr. 25, 2005]).

11. "Public Health Options for China, Using the Lessons Learned from SARS" (paper, WHO China office, July 18, 2003).

3. Joan Kaufman: China's Health-Care Response

1. Board on Global Health, Institute of Medicine, National Academy of Sciences, *Microbial Threats to Health: Emergence, Detection, Response* (Washington,

D.C.: National Academies Press, 2003), http://.nap.edu/books/030908864X/html (accessed May 3, 2005).

2. "Severe Acute Respiratory Syndrome: Status of the Outbreak and Lessons for the Immediate Future," Geneva: WHO: Communicable Diseases Surveillance and Response, 20 May 2003. Accessed on May 3, 2005 at www.who.int/csr/media/sars_wha.pdf

3. Donald G. McNeil Jr. and Lawrence K. Altman, "As SARS Outbreak Took Shape, Health Agency Took Fast Action," *New York Times,* May 4, 2003, A1, 6.

4. Yanzhong Huang, "Implications of SARS Epidemic for China's Public Health Infrastructure and Political System" (testimony before the Congressional-Executive Commission on China Roundtable on SARS, Washington D.C., May 12, 2003). www.cecc.gov/pages/roundtables/051203/huang.php, accessed May 3, 2005.

5. Ibid., 2, Law on Preventing and Treating Infectious Diseases (enacted Sept. 1989), art. 23.

6. Susan Jakes, "Beijing Hoodwinks WHO Inspectors: Hospitals in the Chinese Capital Hid SARS Patients from International Health Officials," *Time,* Apr. 18, 2003. www.time.com/time/asia/news/printout/0,9788,444684,00.html (accessed Apr. 6, 2005).

7. See chapter 4 in this volume.

8. Xinhua, Apr. 2, 2003. www.people.com.cn/GB/shizheng/252/9543/9546/20030402/961472.html (in Chinese; accessed Apr. 6, 2005).

9. John Pomfret, "Doctor Says Health Ministry Lied About Disease," *Washington Post,* Apr. 9, 2003, A26.

10. www.wpro.who.int/chn/docs/Pref_May20.pdf. Accessed on May 3, 2005.

11. Tony Saich and Joan Kaufman, "Financial Reform, Poverty and the Impact on Reproductive Health Provision: Evidence from Three Rural Townships," in Yasheng Huang, Anthony Saich, Edward Steinfeld, editors, *Financial Sector Reform in China* (Cambridge, Mass.: Harvard Asia Center Publications, 2005). Accessed May 3, 2005 at www.fas.harvard.edu/~asiactr/publications/pdfs/huang%20et%20al.pdf

12. Primary Health Care. Report of the International Conference on Primary Health Care, Alma-Ata, USSR, 6–12 September 1978, jointly sponsored by the World Health Organization and United Nations Children's Fund, Geneva: WHO, 1978 (Health for All Series, no.1) and Declaration of Alma-Ata, Geneva: WHO. www.euro.who.int/aboutwho/policy/20010827_1, accessed May 3, 2005.

13. "The World Health Report, 2000. Health Systems: Improving Perfor-

mance," Geneva: World Health Organization, 2000. www.who.int/whr/2000/en/whr00_en.pdf (accessed May 3, 2005).

14. Li Changming, "China's Rural Health in Economic Transition" (presentation to Consultative Meeting of the China Health Development Forum, Apr. 2002, Beijing). www.ids.ac.uk/ids/health/chdf.presentation.ppt. Accessed May 3, 2005.

15. "Guidance for Reforming and Developing Rural Health," State Council Administrative Office, May 24, 2001.

16. Joan Kaufman and Jing Jun, "China and AIDS: The Time to Act is Now," *Science* 296 (June 28, 2002): 2339–40.

17. Gao Qiang, executive vice minister of health of China, presentation at WHO meeting on "Lessons Learned from SARS," Kuala Lumpur, June 17, 2003.

18. The Office of the World Health Organization Representative in China, Beijing, "Public Health Options for China, Using the Lessons Learned from SARS" (unpublished paper, July 18, 2003).

4. Saich: Is SARS China's Chernobyl?

1. On August 16, 2003, Xinhua announced that the last two SARS patients had been released from hospital. A total of 5,327 cases had been reported, with 349 deaths.

2. In fact, the poor handling of information flows led to panic buying as well as rioting and destruction of quarantine centers.

3. For example, when the West Nile virus first occurred in New York City, there was difficulty and controversy in identifying it, including initial faulty diagnosis, and it took around one month to sort out. It also revealed problems of underreporting and lack of knowledge about reporting procedures on the part of the region's doctors and nurses. See "The West Nile Virus Outbreak in New York City (A): On the Trail of a Killer Virus," Kennedy School of Government Case Program, C16-02-1645.0.

4. Hong Kong *Wen Wei Po*, May 8, 2003, trans. in FBIS-CHI-2003-0508.

5. Xue Lan, Zhang Qiang and Zhong Kaibin, "Fangfan yu chonggou: cong SARS shijian kan zhuanxing qi Zhongguo de weiji guanli" (Be on Your Guard and Restructure: Reviewing the Stages of Change in China's Crisis Management from the SARS Outbreak), *Gaige* (Reform), no. 3 (2003): 7–8.

6. Jiang Zemin's "Three Represents" policy asserts that the CCP represents

the development trend of China's advanced productive forces, the orientation of China's advanced culture, and the fundamental interests of the overwhelming majority of the Chinese people.

7. Matt Forney, "How Did a Deadly Virus Find Its Way from Southern China to the Rest of the World?" *Time*, Apr. 21, 2003.

8. John Pomfret, "Outbreak Gave China's Hu an Opening. President's Move on SARS Followed Immense Pressure at Home, Abroad," *Washington Post*, May 13, 2003.

9. See "Incident Resulting from Rumors of an Unknown Virus, Heyuan City Citizens Fight to Buy Antibiotics," Jan. 3, 2003; "Heyuan City Citizens Go to Guangzhou in Panic Buying of Antibiotics," Jan. 5; and "The Appearance of an Unknown Virus in Heyuan Is a Rumor," Jan. 9, *Jinyang Net*. *Jinyang Net* is the online version of the party's *Yangcheng Evening News*. These are quoted in Congressional-Executive Commission on China, "Information Control and Self-Censorship in the PRC and the Spread of SARS," 3, May 7, 2003 www.cecc.gov/pages/news/prcControl_SARS.php (accessed Apr. 6, 2005).

10. Forney, "How Did a Deadly Virus Find Its Way from Southern China to the Rest of the World?"

11. *South China Morning Post*, May 17, 2003. B-type infectious diseases, which allow those infected to be quarantined, include viral hepatitis, AIDS, dengue fever, and meningitis.

12. Pomfret, "Outbreak Gave China's Hu an Opening."

13. See "Guangzhou ruhe kangji buming bingdu" (How Guangzhou Resisted the Unnamed Virus), *Nanfang zhoumo* (Southern Weekend), Feb. 13, 2003. On February 12, the WHO wrote officially to the MOH requesting additional information about the disease, and on February 14, it received written confirmation of atypical pneumonia.

14. Pomfret, "Outbreak Gave China's Hu an Opening."

15. David Lague with Susan Lawrence and David Murphy, "The China Virus," *Far Eastern Economic Review*, Apr. 10, 2003.

16. See "Regulations on State Secrets in Public Health Work, Their Level of Secrecy and Details," in Li Zhidong et al., *Zhonghua renmin gongheguo baomifa quanshu* (Encyclopedia on the State Secrets Law of the PRC) (Changchun: Jilin renmin chubanshe, 1999), 372–74. The regulations were jointly issued by the Ministry of Health and the State Bureau for the Protection of State Secrets on January 23, 1996.

17. As noted above, it was only on February 3 that the provincial authorities had granted it B-type classification.

18. Lague et al., cited n. 15 above.

19. Pomfret, "Outbreak Gave China's Hu an Opening."

20. Ibid.

21. Lague et al., cited n. 15 above.

22. Xinhua, Apr. 2, 2003.

23. John Pomfret, "China's Crisis Has a Political Edge. Leaders Use SARS to Challenge Recalcitrant Parts of Government," *Washington Post*, Apr. 27, 2003.

24. Susan Jakes, "Doctor and Party Member Insists There Are Many More Cases than Officials Will Admit," *Time*, Apr. 8, 2003.

25. Xinhua, Apr. 4, 2003; *South China Morning Post*, Apr 5, 2003.

26. Susan Lawrence, "For the Top, Sorry is the Hardest Word to Say," *Far Eastern Economic R*eview, Apr. 17, 2003.

27. John Pomfret, *Washington Post*, May 17, 2003.

28. Xinhua, Apr. 13, 2003.

29. While in the Shenzhen Special Economic Zone, Hu had ensured Hong Kong's Chief Executive Tung Chee-hwa that he would have Hu's full support in dealing with the epidemic. Xinhua, Apr. 13, 2003.

30. http: www.sina.com.cn, Apr. 17, 2003.

31. The Beijing Joint Working Group for the Prevention and Control of SARS.

32. Xinhua, Apr. 18, 2003.

33. *People's Daily*, English ed., Apr. 21 (http://english.peopledaily.com.cn).

34. This was the committee under Beijing Party Secretary Liu Qi set up on April 18.

35. *South China Morning Post*, Apr. 24, 2003.

36. In fact, in one of her first acts, she drew a long-term foreign resident of Beijing into an informal advisory role.

37. *Financial Times*, Apr. 21, 2003.

38. *South China Morning Post*, Apr. 22, 2003.

39. Xinhua, May 8, 2003.

40. Information from participant.

41. Xinhua, Apr. 26, 2003.

42. Ibid.

43. Xinhua, Apr. 28, 2003. See, e.g., the Xinhua article "We Firmly Grasp

Opportunities in the Time of Danger and Disaster," May 10, 2003, trans. in FBIS-CHI-2003-0510, and the various *People's Daily* commentaries such as "Unswervingly Carry Out Development, the Foremost Important Task," May 17, 2003, trans. in FBIS-CHI-2003-0517.

44. Xinhua, May 14, 2003; *South China Morning Post*, May 15, 2003.

45. Xinhua, Apr. 26, 2003.

46. Ibid. A series of commentaries in the *People's Daily* followed to set the tone. See, e.g., "Forge Ahead Despite Difficulties and Dare to Win Victory—Fourth Commentary on Carrying Forward and Developing National Spirit," May 2, 2003, trans. in FBIS-CHI-2003-0502.

47. Xinhua, May 1, 2003.

48. He also threw in the importance of Jiang Zemin's "Three Represents" for good measure. "Liu Qi Points Out That the 'Double Removal' Marks the Great Triumph of National Spirit," Xinhua, June 24, 2003, trans. in FBIS-CHI-2003-0624.

49. John Pomfret, "China Closes Beijing Newspaper in Media Crackdown. Officials Ban Reporting on Sensitive Subjects, Including Province's Handling of SARS," *Washington Post*, June 20, 2003.

50. *South China Morning Post*, July 2, 2003.

51. *Zhongguo xinwenshe*, May 20, 2003, trans. in FBIS-CHI-2003-0520.

52. *South China Morning Post*, May 9, 2003.

53. *Los Angeles Times*, June 26, 2003. In early September 2003, a Guangdong health official stated that information on infectious diseases collected in a cross-border arrangement with Hong Kong would not be made public. *South China Morning Post*, Sept. 8, 2003.

54. *Financial Times*, May 30, 2003.

55. See Hong Kong *Agence France Presse*, May 30, 2003; *Financial Times*, May 30, 2003.

56. *Zhongguo xinwenshe*, May 31, 2003, trans. in FBIS-CHI-2003-0601.

57. Pomfret, "China Closes Beijing Newspaper in Media Crackdown."

58. *South China Morning Post*, June 13, 2003.

59. Willy Wo-Lap Lam, "Party Bickering Hampers SARS Fight," C:\WINN\temp...\CNN.com-Party bickering hampers SARS fight-May. 13 2003. ht. Accessed May 14, 2003.

60. Pomfret, "Outbreak Gave China's Hu an Opening."

61. *People's Daily Online*, June 11, 2003, http://English.peopledaily.com.cn.

See also Hong Kong *Wen Wei Po*, "The Ministry of Public Security Strikes Hard at *Falun gong* for Exploiting the Epidemic to Spread Rumors," trans. in FBIS-CHI-2003-0509.

62. Kelly Haggart, "SARS and Falun Gong Provide Pretexts for Three Gorges Arrests," Three Gorges Probe News Service, Aug. 14, 2003 (www.three-gorgesprobe.org/tgp/index.cfm?DSP=content&ContentID=8122 [accessed Mar. 27, 2005]).

63. See, e.g., Xue Lan et al., "Fangfan yu chonggou." This is based on a report that was originally presented to the Politburo in mid April on the question of SARS and crisis management. The authors had canvassed quite widely for opinions. Subsequently, Tsinghua set up a crisis management advisory group that included both Chinese and foreign experts and held an inaugural public forum in Beijing on July 18. See Qinghua weiji guanli luntan zai Jing juxing (The Tsinghua Crisis Management Forum Is Held in Beijing), www.people.com.cn, July 19, 2003.

64. Ai Wenbo, "SARS Tests the Government's Credibility," *Zhongguo qingnian bao* (China Youth Daily), Apr. 28, 2003.

65. See Xue Baosheng, "Valuable Lessons for Government to Learn," www.chinadaily.com.cn/cndy/2003-06-06/118111.html, accessed June 6, 2003, and "Cong SARS shijian kan zhengfu xingwei" (Looking at the Government's Behavior from the SARS Incident), in *Zhongguo jingji shibao* (China Economic Times), www.cet.com.cn, May 15, 2003, and "SARS: huanxing guomin xiandai yishi" (SARS: Awakening the National Contemporary Consciousness), www.lsyswy.com, June 13, 2003.

66. Shi Hongtao "China Rebuilding Its Relations with the World During SARS Period," *Zhongguo Qingnian Bao* (China Youth Daily), Internet version, May 21, trans. in FBIS-CHI-2003-0522. The original can be found at www.cyd.com.cn.

67. This was a relatively safe venue. *South China Morning Post*, May 1, 2003.

68. Pomfret, "China's Crisis Has a Political Edge," *Washington Post*, Apr. 27, 2003.

69. Certainly in mid April, PLA hospitals in Beijing were trying to hide the extent of the disease by transferring patients or driving them around during WHO visits. See *Time*, Apr. 18, 2003.

70. Lam, "Party Bickering," May 13, 2003.

71. Interview with relevant Ministry of Civil Affairs officials, Jan. 2003.

72. Xinhua, Oct. 10, 2003. She also complained that many hospitals and lo-

cal disease-control centers had not even downloaded the software that would allow them to report cases of epidemics.

73. Lague et al., cited n. 15 above.

74. In her October comments, Wu Yi referred to the "uncivilized lifestyle" of many localities that laid on big banquets and feasted on exotic animals.

75. *South China Morning Post*, June 4, 2003.

76. *Far Eastern Economic* Review, Aug. 21, 2003.

77. *South China Morning Post*, May 13, 2003.

78. See "Wen Jiabao's Speech at a Seminar on Implementation of 'Emergency Regulations on Sudden Outbreaks of Public Health Incidents,'" Xinhua, May 13, 2003, trans. in FBIS-CHI-2003-0515; and "Wen Jiabao Stresses Enforcement of SARS-Related Laws," Xinhua, May 15, 2003.

79. Wang Dan in *Taipei Times*, Jan. 2, 2003.

80. Of course, as far as we know SARS was an urban phenomenon, but the biggest fear was that the migrant population would spread the infection into the rural areas, thus overwhelming the system. HIV/AIDS offers the same threat. See, e.g., "China: Ministry Issues Circular on Controlling Spread of SARS to Rural Areas," Xinhua, May 8, 2003.

81. *South China Morning Post*, May 7, 2003.

82. See Tony Saich, "The Blind Man and the Elephant: Analyzing the Local State in China," in *East Asian Capitalism: Conflicts and the Roots of Growth and Crisis*, ed. Luigi Tomba, Annali Feltrinelli no. 26 (Milan: Fondazione Giangiacomo Feltrinelli, 2002), 92–96.

83. See, e.g., Xinhua, Jan. 8 and 9, 2003.

84. Xue Lan et al., "Fangfan yu chonggou."

85. *South China Morning Post*, August 14, 2003.

86. Although it must be said that the onset of summer probably also had much to do with reducing the number of infections.

87. Eric Eckholm in the *New York Times*, May 13, 2003.

5. Rawski: SARS and China's Economy

NOTE: The author, who assumes sole responsibility for the contents of this essay, gratefully acknowledges information, comments, and advice from Kam-Wing Chan, David Cowhig, Carsten Holz, Mo Ji, Nicholas Lardy, Guonan Ma, Dwight Perkins, Ruoen Ren, Werner Troesken, and Yifan Zhang, from participants at the September 2003 conference from which this volume originated, and from members of the June 2003 Wianno Summer Study seminar sponsored by the John M. Olin Institute and the Weatherhead Center for International Affairs at Harvard University.

1. Thomas G. Rawski, "What Is Happening to China's GDP Statistics," *China Economic Review* 12, no. 4 (2001): 347–54; Nicolas R. Lardy, "Evaluating Economic Indicators in Post-WTO China," *Issues & Studies* 39, no. 1 (2003): 249–68.

2. Fan Gang writes that with both foreign and domestic investment rising sharply, "we can identify 2002 as the year when China's economy fully recovered from the trough of 1997/98; it is a turning point for genuine positive growth" (*Jiage lilun yü shijian* [Price Theory and Practice], no. 1 [2003]: 13). As is evident from figure 5.1, the official figures show no "trough of 1997/98." Participants in an August 2003 symposium observed that "macro data for the first half of 2003 raise obvious issues that are difficult to explain or even self-contradictory." See "Liuzu tongji shuzi beili, zhuanjia biaoshi jingji jiegou yufa shiheng" (Six Types of Data Show Deviations; Experts Indicate Deepening Structural Disequilibrium) (2003; expired URL accessed Aug. 16, 2003), http://finance/sina.com.cn/g/20030809/1436400009.shtml.

3. Dashan Xu, "High-Tech to Help Build Quality Information Network," *China Daily*, May 16, 2002, 6.

4. See "Roundtable on Chinese Economic Statistics," *China Economic Review* 12, no. 4 (2001).

5. Yunnansheng Shenji Ketizu, "Discussion of Evaluation Methods for Local Party and Government Leaders," *Zhongguo tongji* [China Statistics], no. 5 (2003): 27–28.

6. Nicole M. Christian, "All-out Fight in Detroit to Keep Census above a Million," *New York Times*, May 2, 2000, A18; Juan Forero, "Precinct's Rosy Crime Rate Was Distorted, Police Say," ibid., Jan. 7, 2000, A19; James Dao, "Pentagon Says Lies on Osprey Arose from Pressure to Succeed," ibid., June 30, 2001; Michael Winerip, "A 'Zero Dropout' Miracle: Alas! A Texas Tall Tale," ibid., Aug. 13, 2003, A19.

7. Official data placing GDP growth at 8.0 percent for 2002 cast further doubt on the figures for 1998–2001, which show nearly identical growth rates (fig. 5.1) despite weaker performance.

8. On the (much more severe) influenza epidemic of 1919, see Elizabeth Brainerd and Mark V. Siegler, "The Economic Effects of the 1918 Influenza Epidemic" (2002; http://www.williams.edu/Economics/wp/brainerdDP3791.pdf,

accessed April 22, 2005). Chapter 10 in this volume argues that SARS could indirectly restrict China's economic prospects by limiting the growth of global trade and investment networks, a possibility not considered here.

9. Ren Ruoen, "Feidian bingqing dui 2003 Zhongguo jingji yingxiang de chubu fenxi" [Preliminary Analysis of SARS's Impact on China's Economy in 2003] (MS, June 3, 2003). Professor Ren kindly provided a copy of this unpublished study.

10. *China Monthly Economic Indicators*, no. 8 (2003): 14, 16–17, 29.

11. Dai Yan, "Operations Expect Improvements," *China Daily*, June 13, 2003, 5.

12. Discussion based on information in *China Monthly Economic Indicators*, no. 8 (2003).

13. Yan Meng, "Badly Hit Sectors to Get Support," *China Daily*, May 29, 2003, 6.

14. Xianpu Yan, "Virus' Impact on Sector Should Not Be Overdrawn," *China Daily Business Weekly*, June, 3–9, 2003, 15.

15. Zhongyuan Lu, Liqun Zhang, and Jianwei Li, "An Analysis of the Economic Situation in the First Half of 2003 and an Outlook for the Whole Year," *China Development Review* 5, no. 3 (2003): 2.

16. "China's Economy Not Overheated," *China Daily*, Aug. 9–10, 2003, 4.

17. Dao Wen, "SARS Slows Computer Market," *China Daily*, July 30, 2003, 5.

18. Based on file prc/sars03/bjgdp.083103.xls available from the author upon request.

19. www.sinocheminfo.com/topnews/r200305261013.htm (accessed June 3, 2003).

20. "China May Crude Imports Drop on SARS, Exports Jump," www.hindustantimes.com/news/181_285658,0002008.htm (accessed June 20, 2003).

21. "Chinese Firms Scrambling to Meet Surging Demand," www.google.com/search?q=cache:7nNXZZF2sgEJ:www.oilandgasnewsworldwide.com/bkFeaturesF.asp%3FSection%3D1247%26IssueID%3D268+due+to+expectations+rise+domestic+demand+qilu+zhenhai&hl=en&ie=UTF-8 (expired URL accessed Oct. 10, 2003).

22. Xu Yihe, "China Q3 Oil Products Demand to Rise as SARS Subsides-Analyst," http://biz.yahoo.com/djus/030627/0055000027_1.html (expired URL accessed July 20, 2003).

23. Irene Kwek, "China July Gasoline Exports Seen Up vs Jun; Aug Likely Down," http://biz.yahoo.com/djus/030702/0452000399_1.html (expired URL accessed July 20, 2003).

24. "Gas Exports Down," *China Daily*, Aug. 8, 2003, 7.

25. Other analyses include: Xu Weizhong, "Nine Aspects of SARS' Impact on China's Economy," *Zhongguo wujia* [China Price], no. 7 (2003): 13–15; Yan Xianbo, "Impact of SARS Contagion on Domestic Markets Is Not Easily Overlooked," *Guoyou zichan guanli* [Management of State Assets], no. 6 (2003): 8–10; Zhong Wei, "SARS and China's GDP Growth," *Zhongguo tongji* [China Statistics] 6 (2003): 1.

26. Ren, "Feidian bingqing dui 2003 Zhongguo jingji yingxiang de chubu fenxi."

27. Tranport data from *China Monthly Economic Indicators*, no. 8 (2003): 22–25.

28. Official claims of slowly rising rural incomes draw skeptical comment from Chinese analysts. In 2002, a senior researcher in the State Council's Development Research Centre commented: "The official statistics say that peasants' income is going up, but my opinion, and that of a lot of people that I have spoken to, is that actually their income is falling." An economist from the National Bureau of Statistics noted that rural incomes rose in 2001 "after having been frozen for four years," even though official data show per capita net incomes of rural households rising by 17.0 percent in nominal terms between 1996 and 2000. See *Zhongguo Nongye Nianjian 2001* [China Agricultural Yearbook] (Beijing: Zhongguo nongye chubanshe, 2001), 437; James Kynge, "China's Data Chief 'Confident' About Statistics," *Financial Times* (electronic archive), Mar. 1, 2002; Xianpu Yan, "Rural Market Failing to Spur Domestic Demand," *China Daily Business Weekly*, Aug. 20–25, 2002, 15.

29. Shan Da, "Rural Income Hit by SARS," *China Daily*, July 18, 2003, 7; Bei Xin, "Refilling Farmers' SARS-Hit Pockets," ibid., Aug. 2–3, 2003, 4.

30. Audrey Donnithorne, "China's Cellular Economy: Some Economic Trends since the Cultural Revolution," *China Quarterly*, no. 52 (1972): 605–19.

31. Anjali Kumar, *China: Internal Market Development and Regulation* (Washington, D.C.: World Bank, 1994).

32. Christine Wong, "Fiscal Reform and Local Industrialization: The Problematic Sequencing of Reform in Post-Mao China," *Modern China* 18.2 (1992): 197–227.

33. See, e.g., Andrew Watson, Christopher Findlay, and Yintang Du, "Who

Won the Wool War? A Case Study of Rural Product Marketing in China," *China Quarterly*, no. 118 (1989): 215–41.

34. Alwyn Young, "The Razor's Edge: Distortions and Incremental Reform in the People's Republic of China," *Quarterly Journal of Economics* 115.4 (2000): 1091–1136.

35. Sandra Poncet, "Measuring Chinese Domestic and International Integration," *China Economic Review* 14, no. 1 (2003): 1–21.

36. Genevieve Boyreau-Debray and Shang-jin Wei, *Can China Grow Faster? A Diagnosis on the Fragmentation of the Domestic Capital Market*, accessed Oct. 10, 2003; www.nber.org/~confer/2003/cwgf03/wei.pdf.

37. Sandra Poncet, "A Fragmented China: Measure and Determinants of Chinese Domestic Market Disintegration" (Tinbergen Institute Discussion Papers with number 04-103/2, 2004).

38. Ibid.

39. Thomas G. Rawski and Robert W. Mead, "On the Trail of China's Phantom Farmers," *World Development* 4 (1997): 775; Ralph W. Huenemann, "Are China's Recent Transport Statistics Plausible?" *China Economic Review* 12, no. 4 (2001): 372.

40. Fengbo Zhang, *Zhongguo Jiaotong Jingji Fenxi* [Economic Analysis of China's Transportation] (Beijing: Renmin chubanshe, 1987), 102.

41. *Zhongguo Tongji Nianjian 2002* [China Statistical Yearbook 2002] (Zhongguo tongji chubanshe, 2002), 553, where the number of trucks "used for business transport" is noted as having increased from 124,800 to 4.09 million between 1998 and 1999.

42. *Hubei Gonglu Yunshu Nianjian (1993 Nian)* [Hubei Road Transport Yearbook 1993] (Wuhan: Wuhan chubanshe, 1995), 263.

43. Calculated from standard yearbook data in file \prc\sars03\transport.091203.xls available from the author upon request.

44. Rawski and Mead, "On the Trail of China's Phantom Farmers"; *Hubei Jiaotong Nianjian 2001* [Hubei Yearbook of Transport and Communication] (Wuhan: Hubeisheng jiaotongting, 2002), 536, 554–55.

45. Rawski and Mead, "On the Trail of China's Phantom Farmers."

46. *Hubei Jiaotong Nianjian 2001*, 318.

47. *Jiangsu Jiaotong Nianjian* [Jiangsu Yearbook of Transport and Communication] (Beijing: Zhongguo tielu chubanshe, 2001), 172.

48. *Sichuan Jiaotong Nianjian 2001* [Sichuan Yearbook of Transport and Communication] (Chengdu: Sichuan kexue jishu chubanshe, 2001).

49. Lu, Zhang, and Li, "Analysis of the Economic Situation," 38.

50. See, however, Xinpeng Xu, "Have the Chinese Provinces Become Integrated under Reform?" *China Economic Review* 13, no. 2–3 (2002): 116–33; Chong-en Bai, Yingjian Du, Zhigang Tao, and Sarah Y. Tong, "Local Protectionism and Regional Specialization: Evidence from China's Industries," *Journal of International Economics*, 63.2 (2004): 397–417; Barry Naughton, "How Much Can Regional Integration Do to Unify China's Markets?" in *How Far Across the River? Chinese Policy Reform at the Millenium*, ed. Nicholas C. Hope, Dennis Tao Yang, and Mu Yang Li (Stanford: Stanford University Press, 2003).

51. Guo Xiao, "Develop Bohai Sea Rim Economy," *China Daily*, 4–5 Oct. 2003, 2.

52. www.moh.gov.cn/wsflfg/fl/200205140007.htm (accessed Sept. 3, 2003). Professor Jun Jing indicates that some information about specific categories of infectious disease is treated as a state secret, which indicates inconsistency between laws on disease and secrecy.

53. Tian Mai, "Alumina Business Booms," *China Daily*, Aug. 18, 2003, 6.

54. See www.rediff.com/business/jul/08sen.htm (accessed Oct. 9, 2003).

7. Lee and Wing: Responses in Hong Kong

EPIGRAPH: Rudolph W. Giuliani (with Ken Kurson), *Leadership* (New York: Hyperion, 2002), p. 25, vividly describes the spectrum of emotional responses to public disaster.

1. None of the hotel staff were affected, and it remains unclear how Liu transmitted the infection to so many guests on the same floor.

2. The Prince of Wales Hospital is a major regional hospital that also serves as the teaching hospital of the Chinese University of Hong Kong.

3. It was also uncertain whether the guests of the Metropole Hotel had contracted the virus from the elevator button.

4. Luk Yu Tea House is one of the oldest restaurants in town. It is also one of the traditional establishments that survived decades of modernization and westernization.

5. The Hong Kong government had initially chosen to play down the outbreak. On March 14, Secretary of Health, Welfare, and Food E. K. Yeoh assured the public that there was no outbreak in the community. On March 17, Dr. Yeoh accused the WHO of causing panic over SARS and asserted again that there was no outbreak in the community. On the same day, Professor Sydney Chung of

the Chinese University revealed to the press that there were signs that SARS was spreading in the community, contradicting Yeoh's earlier comment. The next day, Dr. Yeoh admitted that there were SARS cases outside of the health-care workers and their families.

6. Queensway and the adjacent Central District are Hong Kong's financial districts.

7. See also www.cuhk.edu.hk/ipro/pressrelease/030518e.htm (accessed Apr 21, 2005).

8. Emotional disorder was defined using a self-designed criteria. Individuals with four or more emotional or somatic symptoms for four or more weeks were defined as a case.

9. Lee DTS, Sahota D, Leung DTN, Chung TKH. Psychological response to the SARS outbreak (under review).

10. Lee DTS, Wing YK, Leung HC, Sung JJ, Ng YK, Yiu GC, Chen RY, Chiu HF. Factors associated with psychosis among patients with SARS: a case-control study. *Clinical Infectious Diseases*, 2004, 39:1247–49.

11. Wing YK, Leung CM, Kam I: Psychiatric morbidity in severe acute respiratory syndrome (SARS) patients during acute and early recovery stage (under review).

12. Coronavirus had been detected in the cerebral spinal fluid of SARS patients. See Lau K-K, Yu W-C, Chu C-M, Lau S-T, Sheng B, Yuen K-Y: Possible central nervous system infection by SARS coronavirus. *Emerging Infectious Diseases* (online) 2004; 10, www.cdc.gov/ncidod/EID/vol10no02/03-0638.htm (accessed Apr. 21, 2005).

13. See "Bishop and Doctors Stood Up" *Apple Daily*, A12, July 2, 2003.

14. See "Not Purely Anti-23" *Apple Daily*, June 29, 2003.

15. M. E. DeGolyer, "How the Stunning Outbreak of Disease Led to a Stunning Outbreak of Dissent," in *At The Epicenter: Hong Kong and the SARS Outbreak*, ed. Christine Loh and Civic Exchange (Hong Kong: Hong Kong University Press, 2004).

8. Zhang: Making Light of the Dark Side

1. *Beijing Qingnian Bao,* May 16, 2003. http://www.bjyouth.com/article.jsp?oid=2322336.

2. The Chinese term for SARS is *feidianxing feiyan* (atypical pneumonia), the abbreviation for which, *feidian*, is used in many jokes. The English acronym

SARS, which is also used occasionally, is incomprehensible to the general public, and the expansion "Smile and Retain Smile" makes grimly humorous sense of it, at least for those who know some English.

3. Major web sites from which the jokes were collected include www.wellink.net/joke; www.qianlong.com; www.mty.cn/; www.haha356.com; and www.people.com.cn/GB/news/9719/9720/20030509/987752.html.

4. Perry Link and Kate Zhou, "*Shunkouliu:* Popular Satirical Sayings and Popular Thought," in *Popular China: Unofficial Culture in a Globalizing Society*, ed. Perry Link, Richard P. Madsen, and Paul G. Pickowicz (Lanham, Md.: Rowman & Littlefield, 2002), 91.

5. Since the late 1980s, several publishing companies in Taiwan and Hong Kong have published collections of satirical sayings (*shunkouliu*) from China. Some major collections are *Zhongguo Dalu de Shunkouliu* (Mainland Chinese Shunkouliu), vols. 1–2, ed. Gan Tang (Taipei: Research Institute of Mainland China, 1988–89); *Qiwen Guailun Shunkouliu* (Strange and Weird Sayings: *Shunkouliu*) (Hong Kong: Haiyang Zizi Company, 1989); Chen Minsheng, *Cong Shunkouliu Jiedu Xin Zhongguo* (Understanding New China Through *Shunkouliu*) (Hong Kong: Subculture Series, 1997); and Liu Jie, *Laobeixing de Zhihui: Dalu dangdai shunkouliu shangxi* (The Wisdom of the Common People: An Analysis of Mainland Chinese *Shunkouliu*) (Taipei: Mai Tian Publishing House, 2000). In more recent years, some collections have also been published in mainland China: *Baixing Huati: Dangdai Shunkouliu* (The Hot Topics of the Common People: Contemporary *Shunkouliu*), ed. Lu Wen (Beijing: Zhongguo Archival Bureau Publishing House, 1998); *Minyao Xia de Zhongguo* (Chinese Society in Folk Sayings), ed. Nie Ren (Changchun: Shidai Wenyi Publishing House, 2000).

6. Xu Yufang, *Asia Times*, Nov. 6, 2002. www/atimes.com. (Xu Yufang, "The Fading of Jiang's Three Represents." *Asian Times*, Nov. 7, 2002, www.atimes.com/atimes/China/DK07Ad04.html.)

7. Jiang Zemin's "Three Represents" theory asserts that "the CCP represents the development trend of China's advanced productive forces, the orientation of China's advanced culture, and the fundamental interests of the overwhelming majority of the Chinese people."

8. Written by Tian Han and composed by Nie Er in 1932, this song was dedicated to those who rose to defend the nation against the Japanese invaders. In September 1949, the First Plenary Session of the CPPCC passed a resolution adopting this song as the national anthem of the People's Republic of China.

9. "Haoliao ge" ("The Done Character Song," also translated as "The Won Done Song") is a well-known classical Chinese poem, which first appeared in the famous eighteenth century novel *The Dream of the Red Chamber*. The poem's major theme emphasizes that there is no real salvation in the human world and urges people to give up worldly affairs. I thank my colleague Kim Besio for pointing out this connection to me.

10. *Beijing Youth Daily*, May 16, 2003.

11. Xiaotangshan Hospital is a specially designated hospital for SARS patients located in a Beijing suburb. It was built in ten days when many Beijing hospitals were fully occupied and unable to take any more SARS patients or patients with suspected SARS.

12. Ana Club web site: http://bbs12.netease.com/lady/readthread.php?forumcode=10&postid=126692&pageid=2&click_add=n.

13. Alan Dundes, 1987. "At Ease, Disease—AIDS Jokes as Sick Humor," *American Behavioral Scientist* 30, no. 3 (1987): 72–81.

14. In their essay on the overwhelming popularity of *shunkouliu* (rhythmical satirical sayings) in 1990s China (cited n. 4 above), Link and Zhou mention that with the "possible exception of Chinese Central Television and Radio, no medium in China in the 1990s was as widespread as the oral network" of *shunkouliu*. Most *shunkouliu* are social and political satires that circulate "among all strata of society . . . reflecting genuine popular ideas, values, and attitudes with extraordinary vividness" (89).

15. The government's media, such as Renminwang (People's Daily web site) (May 9, 2003), Xinhua News Agency's web site (April 26, 2003), China Youth Daily (April 26, 2003), Liberation Daily (June 2, 2003), and People's Liberation Army Daily (August 30, 2004), all acknowledged the outpouring of SARS jokes, and made positive comments on the phenomenon.

16. Renminwang, www.people.com.cn/GB/news/9719/9720/20030509/987752.html.

17. According to the China Internet Network Information Center (CINIC), the number of China's Internet users grew from 620,000 in 1997 to over 70 million by the end of 2003; see the 13th Report of CINIC in 2003, http://www.cnnic.net.cn/html/Dir/2004/02/05/2116.htm. In 2001, China had 43 million mobile phone users, but by mid 2003, China's mobile phone users reached 234 million; see "The Economic Operation Status of the Communication Sector for the First Half of 2003," the Ministry of Information Industry (2003), www.mii.gov.cn/mii/hyzw/tongji/tongji200301-06.htm.

9. Kleinman and Lee: The Problem of Social Stigma

1. See Erving Goffman, *Stigma: Notes on the Management of Spoiled Identity* (New York: Simon and Schuster, 1963); Arthur Kleinman, *Writing at the Margin: Discourse Between Anthropology and Medicine* (Berkeley: University of California Press, 1995), 147–72; and also papers delivered at the September 5–7, 2001, National Institutes of Health Conference "Stigma and Global Health: Developing a Research Agenda."

2. Arthur Kleinman, "The Background and Development of Public Health in China: An Exploratory Essay" in *Public Health in the People's Republic of China: Report of a Conference*, ed. Myron E. Wegman, Tsung-yi Lin, and Elizabeth F. Purcell (New York: Josiah Macy, Jr. Foundation, 1973), 1–23.

3. On epilepsy, see Kleinman, *Writing at the Margin*. On leprosy, see Zachary Gussow, *Leprosy, Racism, and Public Health: Social Policy in Chronic Disease Control* (Boulder, Colo.: Westview Press, 1989), and Zachary Gussow and G. S. Tracy, "Stigma and the Leprosy Phenomenon: The Social History of a Disease in the Nineteenth and Twentieth Centuries," *Bulletin of the History of Medicine* 44, no. 5 (1970): 425–49. On mental illness, see U.S. Department of Health and Human Services, *Mental Health: A Report of the Surgeon General* (Rockville, Md.: DHSS, Center for Mental Health Services, 1999); and World Health Organization, *Mental Health: New Understandings, New Hope* (Geneva: WHO, 2001).

4. The uncertainty of transmission was especially apropos of the large outbreak at the Amoy Gardens Complex, believed to be due to contamination of the sewage system by a SARS subject with diarrhea, leakage in a skywell, which was a quasi-confined space that facilitated the travel of the virus to upper floors, and dry P traps that emitted contaminated water vapor within the building, resulting in cross-infection of multiple residents. The Government of the Hong Kong Special Administrative Region of the People's Republic of China (HKSAR Government), Department of Health, "Outbreak of Severe Acute Respiratory Syndrome (SARS) at Amoy Gardens, Kowloon Bay, Hong Kong: Main Findings of the Investigation," www.info.gov.hk/info/sars/pdf/amoy_e.pdf (accessed Oct. 20, 2003); World Health Organization, "Environmental Health Team Reports on Amoy Gardens," www.info.gov.hk/info/sars/who-amoye.pdf (accessed Oct. 20, 2003); Andrew N. Baldwin, "Infection Control Within the Built Environment" (paper presented at the "After SARS: Education and Research Agenda for the Future," Joint HKU/CUHK/CPU Academic Seminar, July 2, 2003).

5. Sing Lee, "The Stigma of Schizophrenia: A Transcultural Problem," *Current Opinion in Psychiatry* 15 (2002): 37–41.

6. "One Funeral Home Refused to Handle the Bodies of SARS Victims," *Oriental Daily*, Apr. 1, 2003; Ella Lee, "Epidemic of Fear Spawns Outbreak of Prejudice," *South China Morning Post*, Apr. 12, 2003; "Empty Coffin Placed in a SARS Victim's Funeral," *Sun*, Apr. 30, 2003.

7. "Private Doctors Refused to Treat Suspected SARS Patients," *Hong Kong Daily News*, Apr. 5, 2003; Lee, "Epidemic of Fear"; Michael Ng, "Yan Chai Workers Fear for Safety," *Standard*, Apr. 16, 2003; Patsy Moy and Alex Lo, "Nurse Feels Cheated by Unlucky Draw for SARS Wards," *South China Morning Post*, Apr. 19, 2003; "Doctor with Asthma Fired Due to His Refusal to Work in SARS Ward," *Sing Tao Daily*, Apr. 29, 2003; "Ward Assistants Quit When Deployed to SARS Wards," *Apple Daily*, May 2, 2003.

8. "SARS Patient's Husband: I Lose My Job," *Sing Tao Daily*, Mar. 28, 2003; Lee, "Epidemic of Fear"; "The Family as the Goddess of Bad Luck Because of One Member Infected," *Sun*, Apr. 19, 2003; Niki Law, "Stop Treating Us Like Lepers, Pleads Infected Nurse," *South China Morning Post*, May 2, 2003; Patsy Moy, "SARS Stigma Puts Control of Disease at Risk," ibid., July 29, 2003.

9. "Compulsory Leaves May Become a Mean[s] of Wage-cutting," *Oriental Daily*, Mar. 28; Equal Opportunities Commission of Hong Kong, "Fact Sheet: Role of EOC in SAR Crisis," www.eoc.org.hk/_File/news/FactSheet-e.doc (accessed Nov. 3, 2003).

10. Kar-man Chan, "Services Maintained Despite Virus Attack, Elderly Homes Staff Need More Support," *The Voice*, 309 (Hong Kong: St James Settlement, 2003), http://202.64.132.79/v0309/00002.htm (accessed Oct. 31, 2003).

11. "Residents Nearby SARS Clinics Fear of Infection," *Hong Kong Economic Times*, Mar. 31, 2003; "Those Rejected Medical Check-up Would Be Fired, Companies Asked Employees from Amoy to Take Leaves," *Hong Kong Daily News*, Mar. 31, 2003; "Amoy Residents as 'Monsters'," *Apple Daily*, Mar. 31, 2003; Stella Lee, "Amoy Residents Sent to Isolation Camps," *South China Morning Post*, Apr. 2, 2003; Heike Phillips, "Sai Kung Mother Stirs Fear over Camp's Sewage," ibid., Apr. 4, 2003; "A Man Sneezing Mistreated as a SARS Case," *Ming Pao*, Apr. 9, 2003; Stella Lee, "Bias Body Receives 13 Complaints," *South China Morning Post*, Apr. 11, 2003; "Non-infected Students from Amoy Gardens Discriminated by Fellow Classmates," *Ming Pao*, Apr. 23, 2003; Keith Bradsher, "Now, the SARS Emotional Toll," *New York Times*, June 4, 2003.

12. "Empty Coffin Placed in a SARS Victim's Funeral"; Ella Lee, "Loss of Both Parents Haunts SARS Survivor," *South China Morning Post*, May 1, 2003; Ella Lee, "Angry Son of SARS Victims Challenges Ban on Funerals," ibid., May 9, 2003; "Many Restrictions for SARS Victims' Funeral," *Apple Daily*, May 31, 2003.

13. Lee, "Bias Body Receives 13 Complaints"; Lee, "Epidemic of Fear Spawns Outbreak of Prejudice"; "Doctors from SARS Wards Banned from Departmental Meetings," *Oriental Daily*, Apr. 12, 2003; "Tuen Mun SARS Wards Staff Forced to Take Paid-Leaves," ibid., May 1, 2003; "Empty Praise: Fears of Medical Staff in Public Transport," *Hong Kong Economic Times*, May 14, 2003; "Medical Worker Rejected for Salon Service," *Sing Tao Daily*, May 19, 2003.

14. "Employer Requested Lady Not to See Boyfriend Nurse," *Oriental Daily*, June 3, 2003; "Requested by Boss to Give Up Seeing Boyfriend," *Apple Daily*, May 15, 2003; Bradsher, "Now, the SARS Emotional Toll."

15. "SARS Raised Public Concern about Anti-discrimination,"*Apple Daily*, Sept. 14, 2003; Bradsher, "Now, the SARS Emotional Toll"; "SARS Stigma Stays Despite End of Outbreak, HK Survey Finds," *Straits Times*, July 31, 2003.

16. "Amoy Block E Residents Complain: Imprisonment Better than Isolation," *Apple Daily*, Apr. 1, 2003; "Self-Quarantined Amoy Residents' Fear of Losing Jobs," *Sing Tao Daily*, Apr. 9, 2003.

17. Lee, "Amoy Residents Sent to Isolation Camps"; Kristine Kwok, "More Holiday Camps to Be Used for Amoy Gardens Residents," *South China Morning Post*, Apr. 2, 2003.

18. Bradsher, Keith (2003) "Now, the SARS Emotional Toll."

19. Hong Kong Special Administrative Region Government, "SARS in Hong Kong: From Experiences to Action; A Report of the SARS Expert Committee," www.sars-expertcom.gov.hk/english/reports/reports/reports_fullrpt.html (accessed Oct. 20, 2003), and id., "Outbreak of Severe Acute Respiratory Syndrome (SARS) at Amoy Gardens, Kowloon Bay, Hong Kong: Main Findings of the Investigation," www.info.gov.hk/info/sars/pdf/amoy_e.pdf (accessed Oct. 20, 2003).

20. Data from focus groups in Amoy Gardens conducted by Sing Lee, Y. Y. Lydia Chan and K. H. May Mak on June 12 and 17, 2003.

21. "Nurses: Frontline Troops in SARS Battle Fight Social Stigma," *Singapore Window*, Apr. 6, 2003.

22. M. Y. Chong, "Psychological Impact of the Biodisaster of SARS on

Health Workers" (paper presented at the Asia Pacific Inter-City SARS Forum, Taipei, Sept. 27–29, 2003).

23. Cannix Yau, "SARS Heroes 'left to hurt'," *Standard*, Oct. 27, 2003.

24. Margot Cohen, "Survivor's Life After SARS Is an Onset of New Ordeals," *Wall Street Journal*, Apr. 9, 2003.

25. Trish Saywell, "SARS: Containing the Outbreak," *Wall Street Journal*, Apr. 10, 2003.

26. Erik Eckholm, "The SARS Epidemic: Fear; SARS Is the Spark for a Riot in China," *New York Times*, Apr. 29, 2003.

27. Erik Eckholm, "Illness Brings Subdued May Day in Beijing," *New York Times*, May 2, 2003.

28. "Chinese Villagers Attack Officials over SARS Policies," *Wall Street Journal*, May 5, 2003.

29. Sing Lee, Y. Y. Lydia Chan, and K. H. May Mak, "A Telephone Survey on Perception of the Public on SARS-related Issues: A Joint Project Between the Hong Kong Mood Disorders Center and the Equal Opportunities Commission," www.hmdc.med.cuhk.edu.hk/report/report14.html (accessed Apr. 7, 2005); Moy, "SARS Stigma Puts Control of Disease at Risk"; "SARS Stigma Stays Despite End of Outbreak," *Straits Times*, Jul. 31, 2003;

30. Data from focus groups in Amoy Gardens conducted by Sing Lee, Y. Y. Lydia Chan, and K. H. May Mak on June 17, 2003.

31. Goffman, *Stigma*.

32. Kleinman, *Writing at the Margin*, 147–72.

33. Iris Chang, "Fear of SARS, Fear of Strangers," *New York Times*, May 21, 2003.

34. David Baltimore, "SAMS—Severe Acute Media Syndrome?," *Wall Street Journal*, Apr. 28, 2003.

35. Stephen Smith, "US Allows for SARS Quarantines," *Boston Globe*, Apr. 5, 2003.

36. James Chin, "Global SARS Surveillance: 'Was SARS the wolf at the door or just a mouse that roared?' " (keynote address at the Asia Pacific Inter-City SARS Forum, Taipei, Sept. 27–29, 2003).

37. "Russian Mayor Wants Chinese, Vietnamese Isolated to Combat SARS," Yahoo!News, http://story.news.yahoo.com/news?tmpl=story&u=/afp/20030429/hl_afp/health_sars_russia_030429132841 (accessed Apr. 29, 2003).

38. "Irish Government Requires Hong Kong Athletes to Quarantine Before

Participating [in] the Special Olympics World Summer Games," *Ming Pao*, June 8, 2003.

39. The point has been made that stigmatization may have positive aspects in the case of smoking cessation, but we still insist that a special case would have to be made for its use (Peter Benson, personal communication). See Lawrence Gostin, "The Legal Regulation of Smoking (and Smokers): Public Health or Secular Morality?" in *Morality and Health*, eds. Allan M. Brandt and Paul Rozin (New York: Routledge, 1997), 331–58.

40. Patsy Moy and Benjamin Wong, "Specialist SARS Hospitals Rejected," *South China Morning Post*, Apr. 14, 2003; "Residents Worried about Taipo Hospital Becoming an Isolation Hospital," *Apple Daily*, Apr. 27, 2003; L. Y. Chu, "Proposal of Taipo Hospital as an Isolation Hospital Not Yet Confirmed," *Sing Tao Daily*, May 1, 2003.

41. Eckholm, "Illness Brings Subdued May Day in Beijing."

42. Sing Lee, "A Telephone Survey of Mood Disorders After the SARS Outbreak in Hong Kong by the Hong Kong Mood Disorders Center," www.hmdc.med.cuhk.edu.hk/report/report12.html.

43. Yu, Xin et al., "A Study on Psychological Well Being of Frontline Medical Workers in SARS Wards Using SCL-90," in Proceedings of SARS Conference, Shanghai, Sept. 8–12, 2003.

44. Chong, "Psychological Impact of the Biodisaster of SARS on Health Workers."

45. Mary-Ann Benitez and Stella Lee, "Legal Snag Delays SARS List," *South China Morning Post*, Apr. 11, 2003; Heike Phillips, "The Data They Didn't Want to Release," ibid., Apr. 11, 2003; Geoffrey A. Fowler and Cris Prystay, "Restaurants, Churches, Taxis and Bars Woo SARS Recluses," *Wall Street Journal*, Apr. 25, 2003.

46. Fowler and Prystay, "Restaurants, Churches, Taxis and Bars Woo SARS Recluses."

47. M. D. Su, T. H. Wen, C. C. King, D. Y. Chao, and H. M. Liao, "How Can GIS Help Control Infectious Diseases More Efficiently?" (paper presented at the Asia Pacific Inter-City SARS Forum, Taipei, Sept. 27–29, 2003).

48. See Michael Hardt and Antonio Negri, *Empire* (Cambridge, Mass.: Harvard University Press, 2000); Ulrich Beck, *World Risk Society* (Cambridge: Polity Press, 1999); Michel Foucault, *History of Sexuality, Vol. 1: An Introduction*, trans. Robert Hurley (New York: Vintage Books, 1978).

49. See, e.g., Michael Fumento, "SARS: Post-Mortem of a Panic," www.fumento.com/disease/sarsimpact.html# (accessed Apr. 11, 2005).

50. David Lague, with Susan V. Lawrence and David Murphy, "The China Virus," *Far Eastern Economic Review*, Apr. 10, 2003: 13–15; Susan V. Lawrence, "How to Fail the People," ibid., Apr. 24, 2003: 26–28; Peter Wonacott and Leslie Chang, "Chinese Bureaucracy Blocked News, Failed to Inform Doctors," *Wall Street Journal*, Mar. 18, 2003.

51. Polly Hui, "Health Advice Has Not Reached Us, Complain Ethnic Minorities," *South China Morning Post*, Apr. 3, 2003; Mary-Ann Benitez, "Emotions High as Experts Relived Outbreak," ibid., Sept. 22, 2003; "SARS Report Implies: Hospital Authority May Be Responsible," *Ming Pao*, Sept. 22, 2003; Patsy Moy, "Hospital Chiefs Evading Blame, Patients Group Says," *South China Morning Post*, Oct. 19, 2003.

52. Geoffrey A. Fowler, "The High Cost of Sick Days," *Far Eastern Economic Review*, Apr. 10, 2003: 20; Trish Saywell, Geoffrey A. Fowler, and Shawn W. Crispin, "The Cost of SARS," ibid., Apr. 24, 2003: 12–16.

53. Hong Kong Special Administrative Region Government, "SARS in Hong Kong" (cited n. 19 above); Edgar So and King-wah Lo, "The Prologue of the Outbreak," feature story broadcast on Cable TV, Hong Kong, June 19, 2003.

54. "Nurses: Frontline Troops in SARS Battle Fight Social Stigma."

55. Anna Wu with Sing Lee, personal communication, July 28, 2003.

56. "SARS Survivors Need Help Overcoming Prejudice," *South China Morning Post*, July 29, 2003.

57. "American Chinese Unite to Fight Against SARS," *Wen Wei Po*, May 21, 2003.

58. Patsy Moy, "We Know Where You Live: A Tale of Discrimination," *South China Morning Post*, July 29, 2003.

59. Oliver Razum, Heiko Becher, Annete Kapaun, and Thomas Junhanss, "SARS, Lay Epidemiology, and Fear," *Lancet*, May 2, 2003.

60. T. F. Heatherton, R. E. Kleck, M. R. Hebel, and J. G. Hull, eds., *The Social Psychology of Stigma* (New York: Guilford Press, 2003).

61. Data from focus groups with members of the general public conducted by Sing Lee, Y. Y. Lydia Chan and K. H. May Mak on June 18, 2003; Lee et al., telephone survey, cited n. 30 above.

62. Kristine Kwok, "More Emotional Support for SARS Patients Urged," *South China Morning Post*, May 7, 2003.

63. V. K. G. Lim, "War with SARS: An Empirical Study of Knowledge of SARS Transmission and Effects of SARS on Work and the Organizations," *Singapore Medical Journal* 44, no. 9 (2003): 457–63; Arthur P. Liang, "SARS Community Outreach" (online Powerpoint presentation from Public Health Practice Program Office, Centers for Disease Control and Prevention), www.phppo.cdc.gov/PHTN/webcast/SARSIII/Liang.ppt (accessed Oct. 21, 2003); Barbara A. Govert, "A Public Health Model for Mitigating Fear, Stigma and Discrimination During the SARS Outbreak" (presentation at the 111th Annual Convention of the American Psychological Association, Toronto, Aug. 7–10, 2003); Hiroshi Nishiura, "Mathematical Modeling of SARS: Cautious in All Our Movements," *Journal of Epidemiology and Community Health*, online letter, Sept. 3, 2003, http://jech.bmjjournals.com/cgi/eletters/57/6/DC1#63 (accessed Aug. 30, 2003).

64. Chin, "Global SARS Surveillance."

65. Lee et al., telephone survey, cited n. 30 above.

10. Watson: The Consequences for Globalization

1. Steve Lohr, "Many New Causes for Old Problem of Jobs Lost Abroad," *New York Times*, Feb. 15, 2004, 25. Lynnley Browning, "Outsourcing Aboard Applies to Tax Returns, Too," *New York Times*, Feb. 15, 2004, BU12.

2. John R. Saul, "The Collapse of Globalism," *Harper's Magazine*, Mar. 2004, 33–43.

3. For a counterargument to the one presented in *Harper's*, see Jagdish Bhagwati, *In Defense of Globalization* (New York: Oxford University Press, 2004).

4. Elizabeth Becker, "Staring into the Mouth of the Trade Deficit," *New York Times*, Feb. 21, 2004, B1, B3.

5. Richard Rosencrance, *The Rise of the Virtual State: Wealth and Power in the Coming Century* (New York: Basic Books, 1999).

6. Kevin Kelly, *Out of Control: The New Biology of Machines, Social Systems, and the Economic World* (Reading, Mass.: Perseus Books, 1994).

7. See, e.g., Po Bronson, "On the Road to Techno-Utopia," *Wired* 4, no. 5 (May 1996): 122–26; Robert Rossney, "Metaworlds," *Wired* 4, no. 6 (June 1996): 140–46.

8. Arjun Appadurai, *Modernity at Large: Cultural Dimensions of Globalization* (Minneapolis: University of Minnesota Press, 1997).

9. Ibid., 164–68. On transnationality as a cultural system, see Peggy Levitt, *The Transnational Villagers* (Berkeley: University of California Press, 2001).

10. Aihwa Ong, *Flexible Citizenship: The Cultural Logics of Transnationality* (Durham, N.C.: Duke University Press, 1999).

11. David Harvey, *The Condition of Postmodernity* (Oxford: Basil Blackwell, 1989).

12. See, e.g., James L. Watson, "Virtual Kinship, Real Estate, and Diaspora Formation: The Man Lineage Revisited," *Journal of Asian Studies* 63, no. 4 (2004), 893–910, at 899–904.

13. Margot Cohen, Gautam Naik, and Matt Pottinger, "Inside the WHO as It Mobilized for War on SARS," *Wall Street Journal*, May 2, 2003, A1, A6.

14. Ibid., A6.

15. Ibid.

16. Indira Lakshmanan, "Exploring China's Silence on SARS," *Boston Globe*, May 25, 2003, A3.

17. Donald McNeil, "Most Taiwan SARS Cases Spread by One Misdiagnosis," *New York Times*, May 8, 2003, A10.

18. Joe Sharkey, "Tourism and Optimism Spread in Hong Kong," *New York Times*, Sept. 30, 2003, C10.

19. Wayne Arnold, "Executives in Singapore Chafe at SARS-Related Travel Bans," *New York Times*, May 3, 2003, A6.

20. Jeanne Guillemin, "Bioterrorism and the Hazards of Secrecy: A History of Three Epidemic Cases," *Harvard Health Policy Review* 4, no. 1 (2003): 36–50, quotation from 36.

21. John M. Barry, *The Great Influenza: The Epic Story of the Deadliest Plague in History* (New York: Viking, 2004).

22. "SARS Research Confirms Link to Animals," AP on CNN.Com, Sept. 5, 2003. South China has been perceived (by northern Chinese) as a center of respiratory illnesses for several centuries; see Martha Hanson, "Robust Northerners and Delicate Southerners: The Nineteenth Century Invention of a Southern Medical Tradition," in *Innovation in Chinese Medicine*, ed. Elisabeth Hsu (Cambridge: Cambridge University Press, 2001), 262–91. See also Mei Zhan, "Civet Cats, Fried Grasshoppers, and David Beckham's Pajamas: Unruly Bodies after SARS," *American Anthropologist* 107, no. 1 (2005): 31–42.

23. http://www.cdc.gov/flu/avian/h7n7-netherlands.htm (accessed Apr. 11, 2005).

Index

In this index an "f" after a number indicates a separate reference on the next page, and an "ff" indicates separate references on the next two pages. A continuous discussion over two or more pages is indicated by a span of page numbers, e.g., "57–59."

Printed in the USA
CPSIA information can be obtained
at www.ICGtesting.com
LVHW041125210924
791747LV00001B/29